UNDERGROUND
CLINICAL VIGNETTES

....

OBSTETRICS/GYNECOLOGY

Classic Clinical Cases for
USMLE Step 2 Review [53 cases]

VIKAS BHUSHAN, MD
University of California, San Francisco, Class of 1991
Series Editor, Diagnostic Radiologist

TAO LE, MD
University of California, San Francisco, Class of 1996
Yale-New Haven Hospital, Resident in Internal Medicine

CHIRAG AMIN, MD
University of Miami, Class of 1996
Orlando Regional Medical Center, Resident in Orthopaedic Surgery

JOSE M. FIERRO, MD
Brookdale Hospital, Resident in Medicine/Pediatrics

HOANG NGUYEN
Northwestern University, Class of 2000

VISHAL PALL, MBBS
Government Medical College, Chandigarh, India, Class of 1996

NOTICE

The authors of this volume have taken care that the information contained herein is accurate and compatible with the standards generally accepted at the time of publication. Nevertheless, it is difficult to ensure that all the information given is entirely accurate for all circumstances. The publisher and authors do not guarantee the contents of this book and disclaim liability, loss, or damage incurred as a consequence, directly or indirectly, of the use and application of any of the contents of this volume.

DISTRIBUTED by Blackwell Science, Inc.
Editorial Office:
Commerce Place, 350 Main Street, Malden, Massachusetts 02148, USA

DISTRIBUTORS

USA

Commerce Place
350 Main Street
Malden, Massachusetts 02148
(Telephone orders: 800-215-1000 or
781-388-8250;
fax orders: 781-388-8270)

Canada

Login Brothers Book Company
324 Saulteaux Crescent
Winnipeg, Manitoba, R3J 3T2
(Telephone orders: 204-224-4068;
Telephone: 800-665-1148;
fax: 800-665-0103

Australia

Blackwell Science Pty Ltd.
54 University Street
Carlton, Victoria 3053
(Telephone orders: 03-9347-0300;
fax orders: 03-9349-3016)

Outside North America and Australia

Blackwell Science, Ltd.
c/o Marston Book Service, Ltd.
P.O. Box 269
Abingdon
Oxon OX14 4YN
England
(Telephone orders: 44-01235-465500;
fax orders: 44-01235-465555)

ISBN: 1-890061-23-9
TITLE: Underground Clinical Vignettes: OB/GYN

Editor: Andrea Fellows
Typesetter: Vikas Bhushan using MS Word97
Printed and bound by Capital City Press

Printed in the United States of America
99 00 01 02 6 5 4 3 2

Contributors

. . . .

AMINAH BLISS
UCLA School of Medicine, Class of 1999

NAVNEET DHILLON, MBBS
Government Medical College, Chandigarh, Class of 1997

SONAL SHAH
Ross University, Class of 2000

VIPAL SONI
UCLA School of Medicine, Class of 1999

ASHRAF ZAMAN, MBBS
International Medical Graduate

Faculty Reviewers

. . . .

TAMARA CALLAHAN, MD, MPP
Brigham & Women's Hospital, Resident in Obstetrics/Gynecology

AARON CAUGHEY, MD, MPP
Brigham & Women's Hospital, Resident in Obstetrics/Gynecology

MERITA TAN, MD
Northwestern University, Assistant Professor of Obstetrics/Gynecology

Acknowledgments

Throughout the production of this book, we have had the support of many friends and colleagues. Special thanks to our business manager, Gianni Le Nguyen. For expert computer support, Tarun Mathur and Alex Grimm. For additional copy editing services, Erica Simmons. For design suggestions, Sonia Santos and Elizabeth Sanders.

For authorship, editing, proofreading, and assistance across the vignette series, we collectively thank Chris Aiken, Kris Alden, Ted Amanios, Henry Aryan, Natalie Barteneva, MD, Adam Bennett, Ross Berkeley, MD, Archana Bindra, MBBS, Sanjay Bindra, MBBS, Aminah Bliss, Tamara Callahan, MD, MPP, Aaron Caughey, MD, MPP, Deanna Chin, Vladimir Coric, MD, Vladimir Coric, Sr., MD, Ronald Cowan, MD, PhD, Ryan Crowley, Daniel Cruz, Zubin Damania, Rama Dandamudi, MD, Sunit Das, Brian Doran, MD, Alea Eusebio, Thomas Farquhar, Jose Fierro, MBBS, Tony George, MD, Parul Goyal, Sundar Jayaraman, Eve Kaiyala, Sudhir Kakarla, Seth Karp, MD, Bertram Katzung, MD, PhD, Aaron Kesselheim, Jeff Knake, Sharon Kreijci, Christopher Kosgrove, MD, Warren Levinson, MD, PhD, Eric Ley, Joseph Lim, Andy Lin, Daniel Lee, Scott Lee, Samir Mehta, Gil Melmed, Michael Murphy, MD, MPH, Dan Neagu, MD, Deanna Nobleza, Craig Nodurft, Henry Nguyen, Linh Nguyen, MD, Vishal Pall, MBBS, Paul Pamphrus, MD, Thao Pham, MD, Michelle Pinto, Riva Rahl, Aashita Randeria, Rachan Reddy, Rajiv Roy, Diego Ruiz, Sanjay Sahgal, MD, Mustafa Saifee, MD, Louis Sanfillipo, MD, John Schilling, Sonal Shah, Nutan Sharma, MD, PhD, Andrew Shpall, Kristy Smith, Tanya Smith, Vipal Soni, Brad Spellberg, Merita Tan, MD, Eric Taylor, Jennifer Ty, Anne Vu, MD, Eunice Wang, MD, Lynna Wang, Andy Weiss, Thomas Yoo, and Ashraf Zaman, MBBS. Please let us know if your name has been missed or misspelled and we will be happy to make the change in the next edition.

For generously contributing images to the entire *Underground Clinical Vignette* Step 2 series, we collectively thank the staff at Blackwell Science in Oxford, Boston, and Berlin as well as:

- Alfred Cuschieri, Thomas P.J. Hennessy, Roger M. Greenhalgh, David I. Rowley, Pierce A. Grace (*Clinical Surgery*, © 1996 Blackwell Science), Figures 13.23, 13.35b, 13.51, 15.13, 15.2.

- John Axford (*Medicine*, © 1996 Blackwell Science), Figures f 3.10, 2.103a, 2.110b, 3.20a, 3.20b, 3.25b, 3.38a, 5.9Bi, 5.9Bii, 6.41a, 6.41b, 6.74b, 6.74c, 7.78ai, 7.78aii, 7.78b, 8.47b, 9.9e, f 3.17, f 3.36, f 3.37, f 5.27, f 5.28, f 5.45a, f 5.48, f 5.49a, f 5.50, f 5.65a, f 5.67, f 5.68, f 8.27a, AX10.120b, 11.63b, 11.63c, 11.68a, 11.68b, 11.68c, 12.37a, 12.37b.

Table of Contents

. . . .

CASE	SUBSPECIALTY	NAME
40	Obstetrics	Eclampsia
41	Obstetrics	Ectopic Pregnancy
42	Obstetrics	Hyperemesis Gravidarum
43	Obstetrics	Iron Deficiency Anemia
44	Obstetrics	Placenta Previa
45	Obstetrics	Placental Abruption
46	Obstetrics	Polyhydramnios
47	Obstetrics	Pregnancy with IUD
48	Obstetrics	Puerperal Sepsis
49	Obstetrics	Rape
50	Obstetrics	Reversal of Tubal Ligation
51	Obstetrics	Sheehan's Syndrome
52	Obstetrics	Smoking During Pregnancy
53	Obstetrics	Twin Pregnancy

Preface

. . . .

This series was developed to address the nearly universal presence of clinical vignette questions on the USMLE Step 2. It is designed to supplement and complement *First Aid for the USMLE Step 2* (Appleton & Lange). Bidirectional cross-linking to appropriate High-Yield Facts in the second edition of *First Aid for the USMLE Step 2* has been implemented.

Each book uses a series of approximately 50 **"supra-prototypical" cases as a way to condense testable facts and associations.** The clinical vignettes in this series are designed to incorporate as many testable facts as possible into a cohesive and memorable clinical picture. The vignettes represent composites drawn from general and specialty textbooks, reference books, thousands of USMLE-style questions and the personal experience of the authors and reviewers. Additionally, we present "Associated Diseases" as a way to teach the most critical facts about a larger number of diseases that do not justify an entire case. **The "Associated Diseases" list is NOT complete and does not represent differential diagnoses.**

Although each case tends to present all the signs, symptoms, and diagnostic findings for a particular illness, **patients generally will not present with such a "complete" picture either clinically or on the Step 2 exam.** Cases are not meant to simulate a potential real patient or an exam vignette. All the **boldfaced "buzzwords" are for learning purposes** and are not necessarily expected to be found in any one patient with the disease. **Similarly, the images for each case are for learning purposes only, were derived from a variety of textbooks, and may not match the clinical vignette in all respects.** Images are labeled [A]–[D] and represent 1–4 images of varying sizes, with locations corresponding to a left-to-right, top-to-bottom lettering system.

Definitions of selected important terms are placed within the vignettes in (= SMALL CAPS) in parentheses. Other parenthetical remarks often refer to the pathophysiology or mechanism of disease. The format should also help students learn to present cases succinctly during oral "bullet" presentations on clinical rotations. The cases are meant to be read as a condensed review, not as a primary reference.

The information provided in this book has been prepared with a great deal of thought and careful research. This book should not, however, be considered your sole source of information. Corrections, suggestions, and submissions of new cases are encouraged and will be acknowledged and incorporated in future editions.

Abbreviations

5-FU - 5-fluorouracil
ABGs - arterial blood gases
ACTH - adrenocorticotropic hormone
AFP - alpha-fetoprotein
ALT - alanine transaminase
ARDS - adult respiratory distress syndrome
AST - aspartate transaminase
AV - arteriovenous
AZT - zidovudine
BP - blood pressure
BUN - blood urea nitrogen
CBC - complete blood count
CMV - cytomegalovirus
CNS - central nervous system
CPK - creatine phosphokinase
CSF - cerebrospinal fluid
CT - computed tomography
CVA - cerebrovascular accident
CXR - chest x-ray
D&C - dilatation and curettage
DES - diethylstilbestrol
DEXA - dual-energy x-ray absorptiometry
DHEA - dehydroepiandrosterone
DIC - disseminated intravascular coagulation
DTRs - deep tendon reflexes
DUB - dysfunctional uterine bleeding
DVT - deep venous thrombosis
ECG - electrocardiography
ELISA - enzyme-linked immunosorbent assay
EMG - electromyography
ESR - erythrocyte sedimentation rate
FIGO - International Federation of Gynecology and Obstetrics
FSH - follicle-stimulating hormone
FTA-ABS - fluorescent treponemal antibody absorption
GI - gastrointestinal
GnRH - gonadotropin-releasing hormone
GU - genitourinary
Hb - hemoglobin
hCG - human chorionic gonadotropin
Hct - hematocrit
HDL - high-density lipoprotein
HIV - human immunodeficiency virus
HLA - human leukocyte antigen
HPI - history of present illness
HPV - human papillomavirus
HR - heart rate
HSG - hysterosalpingography
HSV - herpes simplex virus
ID/CC - identification and chief complaint

Abbreviations - continued

Ig - immunoglobulin
IM - intramuscular
INH - isoniazid
INR - International Normalized Ratio
IUD - intrauterine device
IVP - intravenous pyelography
JVP - jugular venous pressure
KOH - potassium hydroxide
KUB - kidneys/ureter/bladder
LDL - low-density lipoprotein
LFTs - liver function tests
LH - luteinizing hormone
Lytes - electrolytes
MR - magnetic resonance (imaging)
NPO - nil per os (nothing by mouth)
NSAID - nonsteroidal anti-inflammatory drug
OCPs - oral contraceptive pills
PBS - peripheral blood smear
PCOD - polycystic ovarian disease
PCR - polymerase chain reaction
PDA - patent ductus arteriosus
PE - physical exam
PFTs - pulmonary function tests
PID - pelvic inflammatory disease
PMN - polymorphonuclear leukocyte
PMTS - premenstrual tension syndrome
PO - per os (by mouth)
PPD - purified protein derivative
PROM - premature rupture of membranes
PT - prothrombin time
PTT - partial thromboplastin time
RBC - red blood cell
RPR - rapid plasma reagin
RR - respiratory rate
STD - sexually transmitted disease
TAB - therapeutic abortion
TAH-BSO - total abdominal hysterectomy and bilateral salpingo-oophorectomy
TFTs - thyroid function tests
TIBC - total iron-binding capacity
TNM - tumor/node/metastasis
tPA - tissue plasminogen activator
TRH - thyrotropin-releasing hormone
TSH - thyroid-stimulating hormone
TSS - toxic shock syndrome
TSST - toxic shock syndrome toxin
UA - urinalysis
US - ultrasound

Abbreviations - continued

....

UTI - urinary tract infection
VDRL - Venereal Disease Research Laboratory
VLDL - very low density lipoprotein
V/Q - ventilation/perfusion ratio
VS - vital signs
VSD - ventricular septal defect
WBC - white blood cell
XR - x-ray

ID/CC	A 28-year-old recently married woman complains of an **offensive vaginal discharge.**
HPI	She states that the discharge is **thin, white, and foul-smelling.** She reports no vulvar pruritus or soreness.
PE	VS: no fever. PE: speculum exam reveals homogenous, grayish-white, watery discharge that yields a **"fishy" odor** (due to volatile amines) **upon mixing with KOH** (= POSITIVE "WHIFF" TEST).
Labs	Vaginal **pH > 4.5**; saline smear reveals characteristic **"clue cells"** (squamous epithelial cells with stippled borders due to adherent bacteria). UA: normal.
Imaging	N/A
Pathogenesis	Normal *Lactobacillus* in the vagina is **replaced by high concentrations of anaerobic bacteria,** including *Bacteroides, Peptostreptococcus, Peptococcus,* and *Mobiluncus* species. *Gardnerella vaginalis,* now recognized as normal vaginal flora, is found in increased concentrations.
Epidemiology	N/A
Management	Treat with a five- to seven-day course of **metronidazole.** Clindamycin is also effective. Treatment can be offered during pregnancy (metronidazole is contraindicated during the first trimester). Treatment of sexual partners is not indicated.
Complications	Bacterial vaginosis is now known to increase the risks of PID, chorioamnionitis, premature birth, premature rupture of membranes, and postpartum endometritis. Patients taking metronidazole should not drink alcohol, as it leads to a disulfiram-like reaction.
Associated Diseases	◼ **Trichomoniasis** Vaginal infection with anaerobic flagellated protozoan; often transmitted sexually; presents with a profuse, yellow-green, frothy, malodorous discharge; motile trichomonads and WBCs are seen on wet prep; "strawberry cervix"; treat with metronidazole.

ID/CC	A 30-year-old woman complains of **vaginal itching, soreness, and an odorless discharge.**
HPI	The discharge is **thick, white, and curdy.** She has a history of **burning on urination** (= DYSURIA). She is taking **OCPs.**
PE	Thick, white discharge present on pelvic exam.
Labs	Wet preparation treated with KOH reveals **presence of yeast cells and pseudohyphae;** vaginal pH normal (4.0); saline smear unremarkable. UA: negative.
Imaging	N/A
Pathogenesis	Factors such as **antibiotic use, pregnancy, diabetes, immunosuppression, and OCP use** can decrease the concentration of lactobacilli in the vagina, allowing for the **overgrowth of *Candida.***
Epidemiology	N/A
Management	Vaginal tablets and creams produce equal cure rates. Treat with an **imidazole such as miconazole or clotrimazole** intravaginally for seven nights or fluconazole orally in a single dose or for three days. Treatment of sexual partners is not indicated.
Complications	N/A
Associated Diseases	◻ **Bacterial Vaginosis** *Gardnerella vaginalis* is the most common etiology; may occur with other anaerobes; presents with a malodorous discharge and vaginal irritation; increased vaginal pH (> 4.5); discharge has positive "whiff" test on KOH prep, "clue" cells on microscopy; treat with metronidazole. ◻ **Trichomoniasis** Vaginal infection with anaerobic flagellated protozoan; often transmitted sexually; presents with a profuse, yellow-green, frothy, malodorous discharge; motile trichomonads and WBCs are seen on wet prep; "strawberry cervix"; treat with metronidazole.

CANDIDAL VAGINITIS

ID/CC	A **56-year-old obese** female is seen with complaints of a nonpainful **lump** in **her left breast** that she detected during routine self-examination.
HPI	Her **mother died of breast cancer** at 56, and her **sister** also has the disease. The patient had an **early menarche,** is **nulliparous,** and still has regular periods (**late menopause**).
PE	VS: normal. PE: 2.5-cm, **fixed, hard, irregular, nontender** mass felt in **upper outer quadrant** of breast (most common site of lesions); **retraction of overlying skin and nipple** (signs of advanced disease); no nipple discharge; left axillary lymphadenopathy; no hepatomegaly or bony tenderness; no neurologic dysfunction.
Labs	CBC/Lytes: normal. LFTs: normal (alkaline phosphatase increases with bone metastasis).
Imaging	CXR: normal (no evidence of metastases). **[A]** Mammo: ill-defined **mass** with multiple pleomorphic linear and branching microcalcifications. **[B]** Mammo: another case with architecture distortion and spiculation.
Pathogenesis	Risk factors for breast cancer include a positive **family history, early menarche, late menopause, late first pregnancy,** nulliparity, obesity, exogenous estrogens, radiation exposure, adherence to a "Western diet," atypical hyperplasia of the breast, and **breast cancer in the opposite breast.** Women with mutations of **tumor suppressor genes BRCA-1 or BRCA-2** are at increased risk of developing breast cancer; BRCA-1 is also associated with ovarian cancer. The inflammatory variety shows angiolymphatic spread and has an aggressive course with early, widespread metastases.
Epidemiology	In the U.S., breast cancer is the **most common malignancy in females** (1 in 9 American women will develop breast cancer), followed by colorectal, lung, and endometrial cancer. The most common variety is the **infiltrating ductal type. Age is the single most important determinant of breast cancer incidence,** with 99% of breast carcinomas occurring after 30 years of age.
Management	A **biopsy** should be done in all cases prior to definitive

CARCINOMA OF THE BREAST

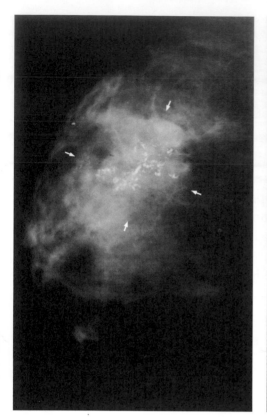 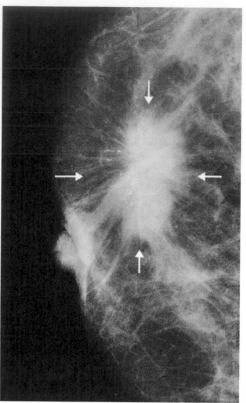

treatment and should be checked for hormonal receptors. Breast-conserving surgery (= LUMPECTOMY) with radiation is the preferred treatment for patients with early-stage disease; modified radical mastectomy offers no advantage over lumpectomy with axillary node dissection and radiation therapy. **Adjuvant chemotherapy** is aimed at preventing late recurrences and usually involves cyclophosphamide, methotrexate, and fluorouracil. **Tamoxifen** may be given alone or with chemotherapy in tumors with positive estrogen receptors.

Complications Infection and/or bleeding of an exophytic tumor, distant metastases, seizures due to CNS involvement, psychological depression, and postoperative local recurrence.

Associated Diseases ▫ **Cystosarcoma Phyllodes** A giant fibroadenoma of the breast with rapidly growing stroma; rarely malignant; presents with a palpable breast mass; mammography reveals neoplasm; treat with wide excision or mastectomy if the size of the tumor precludes lumpectomy.

◧ **Fibrocystic Disease of the Breast** A normal breast variant; patients are usually 30–50 years of age; presents with characteristic micronodular breast texture without discrete lesions; may have menstrual-related breast pain; biopsy shows cystic change, adenosis, and fibrosis; treat with symptomatic measures; rule out malignancy (by mammography and cyst aspiration of dominant cysts); medications used with varying success include progestins, tamoxifen, and diuretics.

◧ **Fibroadenoma** The most common benign neoplasm of the female breast, usually seen in young women; presents with rapid-onset, characteristically round, firm, discrete, movable, nontender nodule in the breast; US shows solid mass; biopsy reveals fibrosis; treat with surgical excision.

ID/CC	A 45-year-old woman complains of two months of recurrent **vaginal bleeding after sexual intercourse** (= POSTCOITAL BLEEDING) and excessive, foul-smelling **vaginal discharge.**
HPI	She has **smoked** two packs of cigarettes a day since age 22. She has been **pregnant five times, first at age 15;** she is a G5P3 TAB2. She has no history of fever, cough, urinary symptoms, nausea, vomiting, or diarrhea.
PE	VS: normal. PE: **emaciated;** speculum exam reveals **ulcerated and friable cervix;** pelvic exam reveals a normal uterus and an irregular cervix that **bleeds on touch.**
Labs	CBC: mild anemia; normal WBC count and differential. UA: normal. PT/PTT and INR normal. LFTs: normal.
Imaging	[A] MR-Pelvis: a sagittal section shows a tumor confined to the cervix. [B] CT-Pelvis: another case in which the cervical tumor has invaded the rectum. Note the bladder (B) and rectum (R).
Pathogenesis	**Human papillomavirus** (subtypes 16,18, 33, 45, and 56), implicated in the pathogenesis of cervical cancer, is found in the transformation zone, where columnar epithelium is replaced by squamous epithelium. Most neoplastic lesions are found at the junction of the squamous and columnar epithelia (= SQUAMOCOLUMNAR JUNCTION). Cervical carcinoma is staged according to the FIGO classification system as follows: 0 = in situ (= INTRAEPITHELIAL CARCINOMA); I = confined to the cervix; II = extension beyond the cervix but not to the pelvic wall (A or B is without or with parametrial involvement); III = extension to the pelvic wall; IV = extension beyond the true pelvis (A or B is with spread to adjacent or distant organs). The tumor spreads primarily by local extension. The most common variety is **squamous cell** (= EPIDERMOID); less common is adenocarcinoma.
Epidemiology	Cervical cancer is the **third most common malignancy of the female reproductive tract** following endometrial and ovarian cancer. It most commonly occurs in perimenopausal women. **Multiple male sexual partners, early sexual relations, HPV or HIV infection, and**

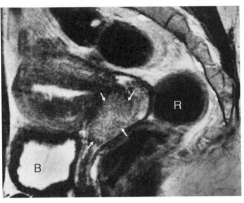 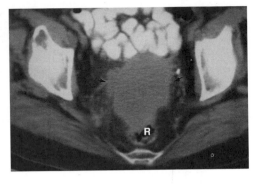

smoking are risk factors for developing cervical cancer.

Management Since the progress of the disease from dysplasia to invasive carcinoma is slow and predictable, and since clinical signs are usually present with advanced disease, emphasis should be placed on **early detection** to improve survival rates. **Pap smear** is the gold standard for screening and should first be performed with the onset of sexual activity. **Colposcopy** and **biopsy** should be done in all suspected lesions or if a large ulcer or tumor mass is seen. No definitive treatment should be instituted without definitive confirmation by biopsy. Cervical cancer is staged clinically by physical exam, CXR, cystoscopy, IVP, and proctoscopy. For **carcinoma in situ,** conization with surveillance is indicated for women who wish to bear children; hysterectomy is warranted if they have completed childbirth. For **stage IA,** extrafascial hysterectomy is indicated; for **stage IB and IIA** a radical hysterectomy or radiation therapy may be undertaken. For disease ranging from **stage IIB to IV,** the treatment includes radiation and chemotherapy.

Complications **Renal failure** (most common cause of death in cervical cancer) from ureteral involvement with hydroureter and hydronephrosis, **hemorrhage** (second leading cause of death), bladder and rectal fistulization, leg edema, and pelvic and back pain due to local extension.

Associated Diseases ◘ **Cervical Polyps** Benign growths; may be pedunculated or sessile; present with prolapse of soft, red lesions through the cervix; may cause postcoital bleeding; treat by removal; can use D&C for sessile polyps.

ID/CC	A 25-year-old woman complains of **vulvar pain, vaginal discharge,** fever, and malaise.
HPI	She was **raped** five days ago and has not had sexual intercourse since that time. She has no prior history of sexual intercourse.
PE	VS: low-grade fever. PE: significant **tender left inguinal lymphadenopathy** (later becomes matted and forms unilocular suppurated buboes or ulcers); pelvic exam reveals heavy, foul, purulent discharge and a few **painful,** demarcated, nonindurated, **soft ulcers** (dirty, ragged edges) **with necrotic bases** in vaginal vestibule.
Labs	Gram stain of pus reveals **gram-negative bacilli** arranged in characteristic **"school of fish"** pattern; culture reveals *Haemophilus ducreyi;* Ito test (intradermal test with *H. ducreyi*) positive; darkfield illumination for treponemes negative; VDRL negative; HIV negative.
Imaging	N/A
Pathogenesis	An STD caused by the **gram-negative bacillus** *H. ducreyi.* Skin trauma precedes infection (*H. ducreyi* cannot invade intact tissue).
Epidemiology	Spread through direct sexual contact (with organism in an open lesion); male-to-female incidence ranges from 3:1 to 25:1. Genital ulcer diseases **enhance HIV transmission;** the association with chancroid is particularly strong.
Management	The patient and the sexual partner must both be treated. In addition to **ceftriaxone,** effective drugs include **azithromycin, ciprofloxacin,** and **erythromycin.**
Complications	Secondary infection and scarring.
Associated Diseases	☐ **Behçet's Disease** An idiopathic autoinflammatory disease affecting young adults; presents with recurrent aphthous ulcers, genital ulcers, and anterior uveitis as well as with rashes and large joint arthritis; treat with systemic glucocorticoids; complications include blindness.

☐ **Genital Herpes** Infection due to HSV-2; spread by sexual contact; primary infection is followed by latency in the presacral ganglia; reactivation is responsible for |

recurrent disease; presents with painful vesicular lesions on the genitalia; Tzanck preparation from lesion shows acantholytic cells with intranuclear inclusions; treat with acyclovir (reduces the duration of episodes and viral shedding but cannot prevent recurrences unless used chronically).

◘ **Lymphogranuloma Venereum** An STD caused by *Chlamydia trachomatis;* presents with tender inguinal lymphadenopathy and painful genital ulcers; inguinal node biopsy is diagnostic; positive immunofluorescence test; treat with doxycycline or erythromycin.

◘ **Syphilis** An STD caused by *Treponema pallidum* infection; divided into primary, secondary, tertiary, and congenital; primary presents with a painless chancre in the genital area; secondary presents with a diffuse maculopapular rash, especially on the palms and soles, and with condylomata lata; tertiary presents with aortic aneurysms, gumma formation, and neurologic disease; congenital presents with fetal death or congenital abnormalities; screen with VDRL or RPR; more specific tests are FTA-ABS and darkfield microscopy; treat with penicillin.

ID/CC	A 22-year-old female presents after recently noticing two nonpainful **"lumps"** on her **vulva and perineum.**
HPI	She denies any vaginal discharge, vulvar pruritus, burning, dysuria, or hematuria. She is **sexually active** with **multiple partners** and does not use any form of birth control.
PE	PE: soft, pink, pedunculated growths 2 mm in diameter; **cobblestoning** of **vaginal mucosa.** **[A]** Another case showing growths in the anal region.
Labs	CBC: normal. RPR nonreactive; cultures for gonorrhea and chlamydia negative; Tzanck smear negative for HSV; vaginal wet mount and KOH negative; diagnostic biopsy reveals papillomatous elongation and parakeratosis with cytoplasmic vacuolization (**koilocytes** are common in HPV infection).
Imaging	CXR/KUB: normal.
Pathogenesis	There are > 70 different subtypes of **human papillomavirus.** Condylomata acuminata are most frequently associated with subtypes 6 and 11, which have little or no risk of causing neoplasia. Subtypes 16 and 18 are associated with premalignant or malignant lesions, including cervical, vulvar, vaginal, and bladder cancer. The virus is transmitted by vaginal and anal **intercourse.** Risk factors include **immunosuppression, diabetes, pregnancy, multiple sexual partners,** and **preexisting vaginitis** (HPV may colonize moist skin).
Epidemiology	HPV is the most common sexually transmitted virus.
Management	Always obtain a **Pap smear.** Urethroscopy may be needed in males with urethral lesions. For small warts, 25% **podophyllin** may be applied locally. Other options include the application of **trichloroacetic acid,** freezing with **liquid nitrogen, laser** removal, **electrical cautery,** and **surgery;** 5-FU and interferon have been used with mixed results. Circumcision may help prevent recurrences in men and their partners. If there is any doubt about the diagnosis or if the lesions do not respond to therapy, an excisional biopsy should be performed to rule out malignancy.
Complications	If left untreated, lesions may become large, necessitating surgical resection. Cervical lesions require monitoring

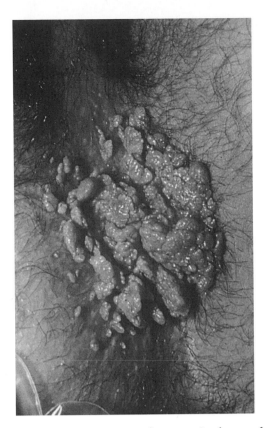

via routine Pap smears for **cervical neoplasia** (although warts do not predispose to dysplasia, coinfection with HPV subtypes associated with dysplasia is common).

Associated Diseases ◼ **Lymphogranuloma Venereum** An STD caused by *Chlamydia trachomatis;* presents with tender inguinal lymphadenopathy and painful genital ulcers; inguinal node biopsy is diagnostic; positive immunofluorescence test; treat with doxycycline or erythromycin.

◼ **Syphilis** An STD caused by *Treponema pallidum* infection; divided into primary, secondary, tertiary, and congenital; primary presents with a painless chancre in the genital area; secondary presents with a diffuse maculopapular rash, especially on the palms and soles, and with condylomata lata; tertiary presents with aortic aneurysms, gumma formation, and neurologic disease; congenital presents with fetal death or congenital abnormalities; screen with VDRL or RPR; more specific tests are FTA-ABS and darkfield microscopy; treat with penicillin.

ID/CC	A **32-year-old** female complains of **menstrual irregularities** and a feeling of **lower abdominal pressure** of four months' duration.
HPI	She is nulliparous and has never used any contraception. Her last menstrual period was one week ago.
PE	VS: normal. PE: well hydrated, thin, and in no acute distress; soft, **rounded, nontender right lower quadrant mass;** bimanual palpation confirms **enlarged right adnexa** with freely **mobile** 7-cm mass located anterior to broad ligament; cervix appears normal.
Labs	CBC/Lytes: normal. TFTs, PT/PTT, and INR normal. UA: normal. Pregnancy test negative.
Imaging	**[A]** CT-Pelvis: an oval-shaped mass (1) with the same density as fat is seen posterior to the bladder (B) and has an area of hyperdensity (arrow) within. **[B]** XR-Pelvis: another case demonstrates teeth within the cyst. **[C]** US-Pelvis: another case shows a mixed cystic (1) and solid (2) mass with areas of calcification (3) due to teeth inside the cyst.
Pathogenesis	Dermoid cysts (= MATURE CYSTIC TERATOMAS) are derived from ectodermal differentiation of totipotential cells and are usually benign. They may contain hair, cartilage, thyroid, nervous tissue, teeth, and skin (three germ cell layers: ectoderm, mesoderm, and endoderm) and may attain a size of up to 20 cm.
Epidemiology	Comprise one-quarter of all ovarian tumors. Bilateral in 15% of cases; affect females in their third and fourth decades of life.
Management	**Surgical removal** of the cyst, leaving a portion of uninvolved ovary if any. Explore the contralateral ovary in view of the risk of bilaterality. Recurrence is rare.
Complications	**Torsion,** rupture with peritonitis, hyperthyroidism caused by secretion of thyroid hormone by ectopic colloid thyroid tissue in the ovary (= STRUMA OVARII), secretion of serotonin (= CARCINOID SYNDROME), and malignant transformation in a small fraction of cases (epidermoid carcinoma).
Associated Diseases	N/A

DERMOID CYST

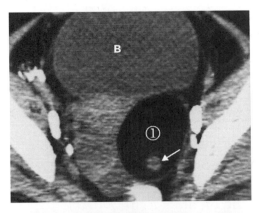
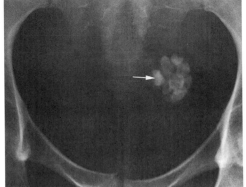
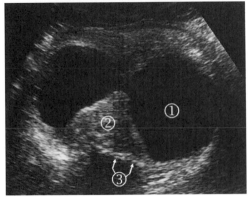

ID/CC	A 21-year-old female complains of a **rash** on her limbs and trunk of four days' duration with **pain** in both **wrists and elbows;** yesterday her left **knee** became **swollen** and is now tender and "hot."
HPI	She is **sexually active.** Two months ago she developed a **vaginal discharge** after several **unprotected** sexual encounters with **multiple partners.**
PE	VS: **fever** (37.8 C). PE: **painful,** nonpruritic **papulovesicular rash** on an erythematous base over anterior and posterior chest and on limbs, with some **pustules on distal extremities** (= ACRODERMATITIS; may also be hemorrhagic or necrotic); rash blanches with pressure; left knee **edematous, erythematous, warm** to the touch, and painful to passive and active motion with restricted range of motion; inflammation and tenderness of Achilles tendons as well as flexor tendons of both wrists (= TENOSYNOVITIS).
Labs	CBC: **pleocytosis** (90,000), mostly **PMNs.** Gram stain (of cervical mucus) reveals **intracellular gram-negative diplococci,** later confirmed by culture in chocolate agar and Thayer–Martin medium; blood culture positive for gonococcus (positive in 50% of cases); throat swab negative; **knee joint tap** reveals abundant gonococci; RPR nonreactive.
Imaging	XR-Knees: effusion with soft tissue swelling; no osseous articular damage (negative in early stage, but may rapidly destroy cartilage and articular surfaces if left untreated).
Pathogenesis	*Neisseria gonorrhoeae* is the causative agent of **arthritis-dermatitis syndrome;** spread from genital infection occurs via the bloodstream (bacteremia). It is typically characterized by painful multiple joints (= MIGRATORY POLYARTHRALGIA) with tenosynovitis followed by a monoarticular (usually knee) arthritis and an acral rash that is usually papulovesicular but may also be hemorrhagic or necrotic.
Epidemiology	Arthritis-dermatitis syndrome occurs much **more frequently in females** and during pregnancy and menstruation; it occurs in 1% of all gonorrheal infections.
Management	**Cultures** (blood, rectum, throat, synovial fluid, skin) are

needed owing to the high rate of false negatives. **Antibiotics** are the mainstay of therapy; administer **ceftriaxone** or spectinomycin with doxycycline for possible concomitant chlamydial infection (50% incidence). **RPR** is needed to rule out syphilis. Sexual relations must be strictly avoided or condoms must be used to prevent spread. It is also important to treat the partner; carriers may be asymptomatic.

Complications

Perihepatitis (= FITZ–HUGH–CURTIS SYNDROME), pelvic adhesions leading to infertility, hepatitis, meningitis, pericarditis, endocarditis, postinfectious arthritis with deformity and persistence of sterile joint effusions.

Associated Diseases

◻ **Meningococcemia** Systemically disseminated infection with *Neisseria meningitidis;* more commonly seen in those with terminal complement component (C5–C8) deficiency; presents with sudden fever, chills, severe headache, meningeal signs, and petechial rash; hypoglycemia, hyperkalemia, and hyponatremia; gram-negative diplococci in blood, possibly in CSF; gross pathology reveals bilateral adrenal hemorrhage; treat with penicillin G, rifampin for close contacts; complications include fulminant adrenal infarction; also called Waterhouse–Friderichsen syndrome.

◻ **Reiter's syndrome** An HLA-B27-associated seronegative spondyloarthropathy seen mostly in males; closely associated with dysenteric infection (*Shigella, Salmonella, Campylobacter, Yersinia* spp.) and STDs (*Chlamydia trachomatis*); presents with conjunctivitis, urethritis, mucocutaneous lesions (circinate balanitis, keratoderma blennorrhagicum), and arthritis; XR shows joint effusion; treat with NSAIDs, doxycycline.

ID/CC	A 17-year-old female is seen with complaints of **prolonged** (> 7 days) and **excessive** (> 80 mL) **menstrual bleeding** (= MENORRHAGIA), **increased menstrual frequency** (= POLYMENORRHEA), and **irregular menses** (= MENOMETRORRHAGIA) for the past six months.
HPI	The patient **denies any breast tenderness** or **lower abdominal pain** (anovulatory cycles). She is afebrile, has no vaginal discharge (making endometritis unlikely), and is not sexually active. Her menarche was at age 14.
PE	VS: normal. PE: chest and abdomen normal; no thyroid enlargement; no signs of hyper- or hypothyroidism; no hyperpigmentation of hands; no leg edema; neurologic exam normal; pelvic exam reveals no masses; uterus normal size; no palpable adnexa or cervical motion tenderness.
Labs	CBC: hypochromic, **microcytic anemia** (due to chronic blood loss and iron deficiency). Lytes: normal. PT/PTT normal. UA: normal. TFTs, LH, FSH, and prolactin normal; pregnancy test negative.
Imaging	CXR/KUB: normal. US-Pelvis: no uterine masses; normal size; no products of conception are seen within or outside the uterus.
Pathogenesis	Dysfunctional uterine bleeding (DUB) is either **anovulatory** (more common) or **ovulatory.** In anovulatory DUB, no corpus luteum develops and progesterone is absent. Unopposed estrogen results in proliferation, necrosis, and random, asynchronous shedding of the endometrium (irregular bleeding). In ovulatory DUB, the corpus luteum develops but does not secrete enough progesterone to stabilize the endometrium (= LUTEAL PHASE DEFECT).
Epidemiology	The most common cause of abnormal uterine bleeding. The two peaks of incidence are **puberty** and **perimenopausal years** (more common). Associated with polycystic ovary syndrome (= STEIN–LEVENTHAL SYNDROME).
Management	After an underlying coagulopathy has been ruled out, **OCPs** or **cyclical progestogens** may be given to regulate menstruation and prevent excessive bleeding on a long-

term basis after acute bleeding is stopped with estrogen. D&C may be indicated for protracted or refractory bleeding. If a patient wishes to become pregnant, induction of ovulation with **clomiphene** may be contemplated. TSH and prolactin levels should be checked to rule out thyroid disease and hyperprolactinemia as causes of irregular menses. **Hysteroscopy and biopsy** are valuable adjuncts in evaluation. Any peri- or postmenopausal woman with a history of abnormal bleeding should undergo **endometrial biopsy** to rule out carcinoma.

Complications Anemia; endometrial hyperplasia with risk of carcinoma.

Associated Diseases ◘ **Endometriosis** Presence of ectopic endometrial glands and stroma; presents with dysmenorrhea, dyspareunia, abnormal bleeding, and infertility; "powder burns" seen on laparoscopy; treat with OCPs, danazol, hormonal control, laparoscopic ablation, TAH-BSO if refractory.

◘ **Endometritis** Infection of uterine endometrium, most commonly associated with delivery and instrumentation; presents with uterine tenderness and fever; leukocytosis; treat with broad-spectrum antibiotics (e.g., clindamycin and gentamicin).

◘ **Benign Leiomyomas** A common estrogen-responsive benign neoplasm of the wall of the uterus, usually in middle-aged women; regresses after menopause; presents with suprapubic pain and cramping, abnormal uterine bleeding, and abdominal fullness, although it may be asymptomatic; US and CT demonstrate the mass; treat with surgical myomectomy; hysterectomy can be utilized if fertility is not desired; complications include severe hemorrhage, degenerative changes (commonly hyalinization and red degeneration), and rarely progression to leiomyosarcoma.

◘ **Endometrial Carcinoma** The most common gynecologic malignancy; associated with unopposed estrogen exposure; commonly presents with postmenopausal vaginal bleeding; diagnosed with Pap smear, endocervical curettage, and endometrial biopsy; treat with TAH-BSO followed by radiation depending on the stage, adjuvant hormonal and chemotherapy for metastatic disease.

ID/CC	A **61-year-old** nun presents with profuse **vaginal bleeding.**
HPI	She reports some **blood loss** with passage of **large clots** a month ago. She has **no pain** but has had significant **weight loss** over the past three months. She is **postmenopausal,** has not had sexual intercourse for many years, and has never been pregnant. She has never had a Pap smear.
PE	VS: tachycardia (HR 110); mild hypotension (BP 100/60); no fever. PE: **obese,** pale, and ill-looking; atrophic vulva; speculum exam reveals old blood in cervical canal and vagina; uterus **enlarged but mobile; no adnexal swelling;** cervix patulous; clot seen protruding from os; uterine cavity D&C confirmed a wide, expanded cavity; **necrotic tumor obtained from all surfaces; curettage provoked heavy bleeding** and patient received three units of blood.
Labs	CBC: **normocytic, normochromic anemia** (blood loss). Pap smear reveals atrophic tissue; endocervical curettage reveals **no tumor;** endometrial curettage reveals **poorly differentiated adenocarcinoma** with invasion into underlying myometrium and extensive necrosis.
Imaging	US-Pelvis: uniformly **enlarged uterus; cavity expanded** and contained echoes consistent with blood clot and debris; no ovarian enlargement. US-Transvaginal: endometrial thickness > 8 cm. **[A]** CT-Pelvis: another case showing an irregular uterine mass between the bladder (B) and rectum (R).
Pathogenesis	A neoplastic disease **of unknown etiology.** Most women have a history of **unopposed estrogen exposure;** however, endometrial carcinoma may develop in patients (especially older patients) without endometrial hyperplasia. Other risk factors include **obesity, nulliparity, diabetes**, and **late menopause.** The tumor is spread primarily by direct extension to the cervix and myometrium and via the lymphatics to the adnexa and peritoneal cavity.
Epidemiology	Endometrial carcinoma is the **most common malignancy of the female genital tract** and the fourth most common cancer in females; 1 in 50 women in the U.S. will develop this disease. It primarily occurs in

ENDOMETRIAL CARCINOMA

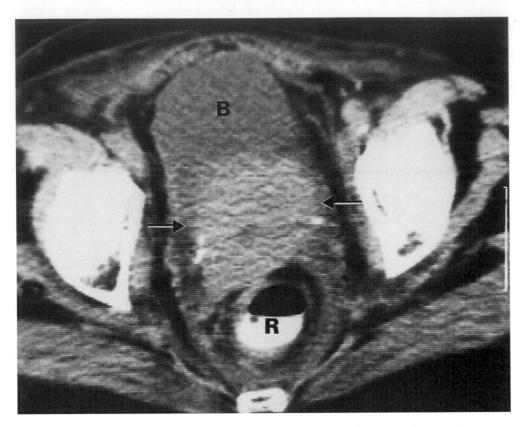

women 50–65 years of age. Adenocarcinoma is the most common type.

Management   For **stage I disease,** where cancer is limited to the corpus, a total abdominal hysterectomy and bilateral salpingo-oophorectomy or radical hysterectomy will suffice; **stage II disease,** in which the cancer has involved the corpus and the cervix, is treated with preoperative intracavitary radiotherapy followed by abdominal hysterectomy, bilateral salpingo-oophorectomy, and pelvic node dissection (this is followed by radiotherapy if the nodes are found to be involved). For **stage III disease,** in which the cancer has extended outside the uterus but not outside the true pelvis, a combination of radiotherapy and chemotherapy (with progesterone) is employed; surgery in these cases is hazardous and may be attempted after pretreatment with radiotherapy. For **stage IV,** in which the cancer has spread outside the true pelvis (to either adjacent or distant organs), progestogens and multidrug chemotherapy are used to contribute to longevity; vaginal metastases may be locally excised, pulmonary metastases are responsive to progestogen, and brain and bone metastases respond to radiotherapy.

Complications   N/A

Associated Diseases   ◨ **Atrophic Vaginitis** Results from estrogen withdrawal (e.g., menopause); presents with dyspareunia, white discharge (= LEUKORRHEA), pruritus, and punctate vaginal mucosal hemorrhages; treat with topical estrogen.

ID/CC	A 27-year-old female complains of **inability to conceive** for four years.
HPI	The patient has had **chronic pelvic pain** for eight years with an **increase in the quantity and frequency of her menstrual periods** (= HYPERPOLYMENORRHEA). She has also experienced progressively worsening **dysmenorrhea** and **pain during coitus** (= DYSPAREUNIA).
PE	VS: mild hypotension (BP 100/60); no fever. PE: umbilical area shows 3-mm **hyperpigmented, raised, nontender nodule** (extrapelvic endometrial implant); pelvic exam reveals **fixed, retroverted uterus** with **uterosacral ligament nodularity;** cervix normal; diagnostic laparoscopy reveals multiple rust-colored (= "POWDER BURN") endometrial implants in ovaries, round and broad ligaments, tubes, and cul-de-sac with adhesions.
Labs	CBC/Lytes: normal. TFTs normal. UA: normal. Infertility panel normal in patient and spouse; biopsies (of endometrial implants) reveal **stroma and glands** identical to endometrium (diagnostic of endometriosis).
Imaging	CXR: normal. US-Abdomen: cystic masses in both ovaries.
Pathogenesis	**Abnormal implantation of endometrial tissue** outside the uterine cavity, leading to infertility, dyspareunia, and dysmenorrhea. Endometriomas (= CHOCOLATE CYSTS) may also be seen, as may hematuria with bladder involvement or rectal bleeding with rectal involvement. It most commonly affects the **ovaries bilaterally.** The diagnosis can be made only by visual inspection of the abdomen (laparoscopy or laparotomy).
Epidemiology	Mean age of presentation is 27, but incidence is not linked to age, race, or socioeconomic status. If present in older children or teens, it can be due to a defect in müllerian duct development. A **family history** of the disease, **retrograde menstruation,** and a history of **prolonged hyperpolymenorrhea** have all been associated with an increased risk of developing symptomatic endometriosis. Approximately 10% of women will develop endometriosis.

11.   **ENDOMETRIOSIS**

Management	The first line of treatment is usually NSAIDs in conjunction with OCPs given in a continuous fashion (i.e., no placebo pills are taken) to suppress stimulation and growth of endometrial implants. More aggressive endometriosis may be managed with Depo-Provera (IM progesterone), Lupron (a GnRH analog), or danazol (an androgen derivative). **Surgical measures** include laparoscopic coagulation, laser ablation of lesions, or open surgery with removal of lesions and freeing of adhesions. In cases involving chronic pain that is refractory to medical treatment, a **total hysterectomy with bilateral salpingo-oophorectomy** may be required. In some patients, a **medical and surgical** approach is needed for long-term pain relief.
Complications	Disabling pain, infertility that is refractory to treatment, and recurrent disease when an ovary is preserved after hysterectomy.
Associated Diseases	◻ **Dysfunctional Uterine Bleeding** Usually due to anovulation, often near menarche or menopause; presents with menstrual irregularities; treat with estrogen and progesterone.

◻ **Pelvic Inflammatory Disease** A polymicrobial infection of the upper genital tract ascending from the lower genital tract, usually due to STDs caused by *Neisseria gonorrhoeae* and *Chlamydia trachomatis;* presents with lower abdominal pain and adnexal tenderness with vaginal discharge; leukocytosis with left shift; high vaginal and cervical swabs may yield organism; treat with cefoxitin and doxycycline; complications include tubo-ovarian abscess, peritonitis, ectopic pregnancy, and infertility.

◻ **Benign Leiomyomas** A common estrogen-responsive benign neoplasm of the wall of the uterus, usually in middle-aged women; regresses after menopause; presents with suprapubic pain and cramping, abnormal uterine bleeding, and abdominal fullness, although it may be asymptomatic; US and CT demonstrate the mass; treat with surgical myomectomy; hysterectomy can be utilized if fertility is not desired; complications include severe hemorrhage, degenerative changes (commonly |

hyalinization and red degeneration), and rarely progression to leiomyosarcoma.

ID/CC	An 18-year-old G1P0 at 20 weeks' gestation presents with **irregular vaginal bleeding** and **mild abdominal pain.**
HPI	She also complains of **excessive nausea and vomiting** (hyperemesis), anxiety, tremulousness (hyperthyroid features), and swelling of her hands, face, and feet. A home **pregnancy test was positive.** She has been **amenorrheic for 20 weeks** but has not felt any **fetal movements;** she has at times noted the passage of grape-shaped **vesicles** vaginally. This is her first pregnancy; she denies having attempted an abortion.
PE	VS: **hypertension** (BP 145/90); **tachycardia** (HR 105). PE: appears pale and ill; bilateral pitting pedal edema present; fine tremor of hands; abdominal exam reveals that **fundal height** (24 weeks) **is more than expected** (20 weeks); uterus feels doughy in consistency (due to absence of amniotic fluid); **fetal heart not heard with doppler.**
Labs	CBC: normocytic, normochromic anemia. UA: proteinuria. Elevated T3 and T4; **serum beta-hCG extremely high** (> 100,000) relative to the expected value; **serum human placental lactogen very low;** histopathologic exam of tissue obtained after uterine evacuation reveals 1–2 L of a **stringy mass of swollen villi without fetal parts;** microscopy reveals **hydropic villi without blood vessels and a minor trophoblast component** (more trophoblastic tissue indicates invasive mole).
Imaging	US-Pelvis: "snowstorm" appearance in the uterus and absence of fetal shadow; presence of bilateral **theca-lutein cysts** in the ovaries. XR-Chest (done to rule out any metastases): normal.
Pathogenesis	**Complete moles** (46, XX) contain no fetal parts, are paternally derived, are associated with symptoms of preeclampsia, hyperemesis, and thyrotoxicosis, and have a **high potential to become invasive or to develop into a choriocarcinoma. Partial moles** (69, XXY; 69, XYY) contain fetal parts, are maternally and paternally derived, and have a **low malignant potential.** A previous molar pregnancy places the patient at risk for future molar pregnancies.

HYDATIDIFORM MOLE

Epidemiology	Gestational trophoblastic neoplasia is a spectrum of disorders involving the abnormal proliferation of trophoblastic (= PLACENTAL) tissue. This includes hydatidiform moles (80%), invasive moles (10%–15%), choriocarcinoma (2%–5%), and placental-site trophoblastic tumor (rare). In the U.S., the incidence of molar pregnancy is 1 in 1,000 pregnancies. Invasive disease develops in 10% of cases; choriocarcinoma develops in 2% of moles.
Management	**Immediate removal** of uterine contents; **follow up hCG levels to detect development of invasive mole or choriocarcinoma.** Pelvic exam for any cervical/vaginal metastases and regression of ovarian cysts, chest x-ray to identify pulmonary metastases, and diagnostic curettage if bleeding persists. **Pregnancy is discouraged** during the follow-up period to prevent interference with diagnostic assaying of hCG levels. Treatment of **nonmetastatic disease consists of single-agent chemotherapy** using either methotrexate or actinomycin D; treatment of **metastatic disease** involves use of either **single-agent or multiple-agent regimens** (methotrexate, actinomycin D, chlorambucil), depending on the prognosis. Malignant forms of the disease (both invasive moles and choriocarcinoma) are exquisitely sensitive to chemotherapy. Radiotherapy may be used for brain and liver metastases. **Hysterectomy** is an option in women who have completed childbearing.
Complications	Metastatic disease involving lung, liver, and brain.
Associated Diseases	◼ **Hyperemesis Gravidarum** An idiopathic disorder of pregnancy associated with hydatidiform mole; presents with refractory nausea and vomiting that interferes with nutrition; usually resolves by the second trimester; may be associated with elevated hCG; treat with antiemetics and hydration; rule out hydatidiform mole by US.

ID/CC	A 32-year-old female is referred to a clinic for **inability to conceive.**
HPI	The patient was married two years ago, has not used any form of contraception, and has had unprotected sexual intercourse at least twice a week. She had a therapeutic **abortion seven years ago** and has noted **irregular bleeding** since that time. She denies any other medical or surgical history.
PE	VS: normal. PE: thyroid not palpable; no breast masses, retractions, or secretion from nipple; abdomen soft and nontender; uterus not palpable; no skin rashes (rules out lupus); pelvic exam reveals uterus of normal size with regular surface, no masses, and no pain on cervical motion; adnexa not palpable; cervix appears normal; normal visual fields (decreases likelihood of pituitary involvement).
Labs	CBC/Lytes/UA: normal. TFTs normal; cortisol, prolactin, testosterone, and DHEA levels normal.
Imaging	CXR/KUB: normal. US-Abdomen and Pelvis: intrauterine adhesions between the two inner walls of the endometrial cavity; no adnexal masses.
Pathogenesis	Infertility is defined as the **inability to conceive for one year after regular unprotected sexual intercourse.** The most common cause of infertility is **lack of normal spermatogenesis; lack of ovulatory cycles** and **anatomic defects** of the female genitalia are also implicated. Causes of **male infertility** include mumps orchitis with atrophy, antisperm antibodies, Klinefelter's syndrome, retrograde ejaculation, varicocele, hypogonadotropic hypogonadism, and Sertoli-cell-only syndrome. **Anatomic abnormalities** involved include congenital defects; acquired defects such as **Asherman's syndrome,** which consists of intrauterine adhesions (= SYNECHIAE) due to previous vigorous curettage of intrauterine infection; **PID,** which produces adhesions that may obstruct the fallopian tubes; **leiomyomata;** and **endometriosis.**
Epidemiology	Infertility affects 15% of married couples with wives of childbearing age. In 10% of cases, infertility is idiopathic.
Management	Measure luteal phase **progesterone levels** and **basal**

body temperature (shows a biphasic curve in women who ovulate, with a peak temperature seen in consonance with the rise in progesterone following LH surge; during menstruation, temperature goes back down) to ascertain ovulation. Patients who complain of fullness of the breasts and lower abdominal/back discomfort and who have regular menstrual cycles are more likely to have regular ovulatory cycles. **Endometrial biopsy** and **urine LH levels** similarly aid in diagnosing luteal phase defects and ovulation, respectively. **Hysterosalpingography** can show the endometrial cavity and tubes, and **laparoscopy** is very helpful in diagnosing endometriosis and adhesion formation. Normal **semen analysis** (sample taken after 48 hours of abstinence) shows a volume of more than 3 mL, with a minimum of 20 million sperms/mL; normal motility entails 50% of sperms with forward motion. More than 60% of sperm should be morphologically normal, and there must be < 1 million WBCs/mL. More than 75% of infertile couples eventually conceive with treatment. Treatment varies according to the cause and ranges from induction of ovulation with **clomiphene** or gonadotropins to surgical correction of anatomic abnormalities, in vitro fertilization, and artificial insemination.

Complications

Depression, anxiety, disruption of family life, and multiple-gestation pregnancies after induction of ovulation.

Associated Diseases

◘ **Endometriosis** Presence of ectopic endometrial glands and stroma; presents with dysmenorrhea, dyspareunia, abnormal bleeding, and infertility; "powder burns" seen on laparoscopy; treat with OCPs, danazol, hormonal control, laparoscopic ablation, TAH-BSO if refractory.

ID/CC	A **40-year-old** woman complains of **blood-stained discharge** from the left nipple; she is concerned that she may have breast cancer.
HPI	She reports a **small lump beneath the areola** of her left breast. She has no other lumps in her breasts or axillae and no family history of breast cancer.
PE	VS: normal. PE: **serosanguineous discharge** from left nipple **and small cystic** swelling beneath areola; **no nipple retraction;** no other breast lumps or axillary lymphadenopathy; right breast normal.
Labs	Tissue removed after microdochectomy reveals intraductal papilloma. Cytology of nipple discharge is neither cost-effective nor reliable, since the risk of malignancy is so low.
Imaging	Mammo: no other pathology.
Pathogenesis	**The most common cause of unilateral blood-stained discharge from the nipple.** Although generally a **single papilloma** in a lactiferous duct, multiple benign lesions may occur. Spontaneous clear, watery, or serosanguineous nipple discharge from a single duct has less than a 7% chance of being malignant.
Epidemiology	The condition is **rare before the age of 25** and usually occurs in women between the ages of 35 and 50.
Management	**Microdochectomy** is the preferred treatment; however, if the duct of origin of nipple bleeding cannot be identified or when bleeding is occurring from many ducts, **cone excision** of the major duct system may be undertaken.
Complications	N/A
Associated Diseases	◼ **Paget's Disease of the Breast** Aggressive breast cancer with overlying skin erythema; presents with itching, burning, and discharge; superficial erosion and eczematous scaling may be apparent; biopsy shows "Paget cells" invading the dermis; requires surgical excision.

ID/CC	A **51-year-old** woman complains of **hot flashes, night sweats, and emotional lability.**
HPI	She also notes **decreased libido, painful coitus** (= DYSPAREUNIA) due to decreased vaginal lubrication, and **painful micturition** (= DYSURIA). She began menopause one year ago.
PE	Gynecologic exam reveals **atrophic vaginitis.**
Labs	**Elevated FSH and LH; cholesterol and triglycerides increased** in relation to premenopausal levels (decreased HDL and increased LDL and VLDL).
Imaging	CXR-Spine: **osteoporotic bone.**
Pathogenesis	Menopause is the cessation of menstrual periods due to a decline in estrogen and progesterone production from the ovaries. The peripheral conversion of adrenal androstenedione to estrogen becomes the principal source of estrogen after menopause.
Epidemiology	The average age of menopause in Western societies is **51 years.**
Management	**Estrogen-progesterone therapy** in women in whom the uterus is still present; give unopposed continuous estrogen therapy in women who have had a hysterectomy (**unopposed estrogen therapy increases the risk of endometrial cancer** by inducing atypical adenomatous hyperplasia). **Calcium supplementation** and weight-bearing exercises should be prescribed for prevention of osteoporosis.
Complications	**Atrophic vulvovaginitis, atrophic trigonitis (bladder) and urethritis, ischemic heart disease** (due to an unfavorable lipid profile), pelvic relaxation, and **osteoporosis.**
Associated Diseases	◼ **Osteoporosis** Quantitative reduction of total skeletal bone mass due to increased bone resorption; usually seen in postmenopausal women (preventable with postmenopausal estrogen replacement); commonly presents with spinal compression fractures, wrist fractures, hip fractures, or acquired kyphosis; DEXA scan reveals diminished bone density; XRs of the spine may reveal kyphosis and osteoporotic collapse of mid- to lower thoracic and lumbar vertebrae; treat with calcium

supplements, estrogen, bisphosphonates, and exercise; complications include fractures.

ID/CC	A **38-year-old** woman presents with **left-sided weakness** and **numbness.**
HPI	She is **hypertensive, obese,** and a **chronic smoker** who occasionally has **migraines;** she has been **taking OCPs** for approximately four years.
PE	VS: hypertension (BP 145/90). PE: pupils equal, round, and reactive to light and accommodation; cranial nerves intact; left arm and leg show **2/5 strength, increased tone, and exaggerated reflexes; decreased pain sensation** on left side.
Labs	CBC: increased hematocrit and hemoglobin (chronic smoker). **Cholesterol and triglycerides** markedly increased.
Imaging	CT-Head: **right-sided infarct;** no areas of hemorrhage.
Pathogenesis	**Cerebrovascular accidents (CVAs), DVT,** and **pulmonary embolism** are more common in OCP users than in nonusers. This may be due to intimal and medial vascular injury, increased platelet aggregation, and a decrease in antithrombin III activity and plasminogen activator caused by the estrogen component of the pill. The effect is dose dependent; with reduction in the estrogen content of the pill, the incidence of thromboembolic disorders falls.
Epidemiology	Other predisposing factors include **age > 35 years, blood group other than O,** heavy **smoking, hypertension, diabetes,** migraine, and **hyperlipidemia.**
Management	Discontinue OCPs. **Heparinize** after ruling out bleeding with head CT and fecal occult blood. **Fluid restriction** and corticosteroids to prevent cerebral edema. Long-term **physiotherapy.** Where applicable, counsel the patient to stop smoking.
Complications	Side effects of birth control pill use (related mainly to the estrogen component) include **pulmonary embolism, vaginal spotting, depression,** breast engorgement, malignant hypertension, hepatic adenomas, nausea, weight gain, cholestasis, amenorrhea or hypomenorrhea, and decreased glucose tolerance. OCPs are contraindicated in women who are > 35 years and

OCP-RELATED CEREBROVASCULAR ACCIDENT

smoke > 15 cigarettes a day; those who have a history of thromboembolic disease; those who have concurrent breast or endometrial cancer; and those who have completed a term pregnancy within 10–14 days.

Associated Diseases   N/A

OCP-RELATED CEREBROVASCULAR ACCIDENT

ID/CC	A **58-year-old** woman is found to have a **pelvic mass** during a routine yearly physical examination.
HPI	She is diabetic and hypertensive and has been complaining of **vague GI symptoms,** including diarrhea alternating with constipation. She has recently been feeling **lower abdominal heaviness** and notes **increasing abdominal girth.** She denies any postmenopausal bleeding or weight loss.
PE	VS: normal. PE: no acute distress; abdomen firm and nontender; ascites present; **mass felt** in left iliac fossa (in postmenopausal women, regarded as **malignant until proven otherwise**); no peritoneal signs; pelvic examination confirms **left fixed, nontender adnexal mass;** cervix normal; rectal exam normal.
Labs	CBC: mild anemia; no leukocytosis. Lytes: normal. **CA-125 elevated** (> 35; also elevated in endometriosis, fibroids, and PID). LFTs: normal. Blood glucose normal. UA: normal.
Imaging	CXR: normal. CT/US-Pelvis: cystic mass 6 cm in diameter with solid areas in the left ovary; omental caking; ascites.
Pathogenesis	Ovarian carcinoma often attains considerable size before it is detected; nearly 75% of cases have **metastases at diagnosis.** Of all ovarian cancers, 90% are epithelial in origin. Of these, the most common variety is **serous cystadenocarcinoma** (may also be mucinous); other types include solid endometrioid carcinomas and Brenner's tumors. Twenty percent of ovarian cancers are derived from the germ cell of the ovary (e.g., teratomas, dysgerminomas); 10% originate from the ovarian stroma (e.g., fibromas, granulosa-theca cell tumors). Ovarian cancer is staged surgically; according to FIGO staging, **stage I** is confined to the ovaries, **stage II** involves pelvic extension, **stage III** involves intraperitoneal and lymph node metastases, and **stage IV** shows distant metastases. Ovarian carcinoma spreads **lymphatically** to the regional nodes **directly** through peritoneal seeding and **hematogenously** to the **liver, bone,** and **lungs.** Carcinoma of the ovary is not always primary; metastases from the stomach (= KRUKENBERG TUMOR), breast, and colon are seen in 5%–10% of cases.

Epidemiology	Ovarian cancer is the **second most common cancer** of the female reproductive tract and the **leading cause of death from gynecologic cancer** in the U.S., showing an overall five-year survival rate of about 15%. Its highest incidence is in women between the ages of 40 and 65. A **family history** of ovarian cancer, **nulliparity, delayed childbirth,** and **late age at menopause** are strong predisposing factors. OCPs have been shown to decrease the risk of ovarian cancer. Women with breast cancer have a twofold increase in ovarian cancer.
Management	**Total abdominal hysterectomy** with **bilateral salpingo-oophorectomy,** omentectomy, and lymphadenectomy if the tumor is in its early stages. If resection is not possible, an attempt is made to debulk the tumor so that the remaining lesion is < 2 cm. **Chemotherapy** (platinum-based chemotherapy and taxol) and/or **radiotherapy** may then be employed with a second-look laparotomy or laparoscopy at a later date. Peritoneal washings, para-aortic nodes, diaphragmatic biopsy, and omentum are taken as specimens for staging purposes at the time of the first surgical exploration.
Complications	Ascites, pelvic pain, anemia, wasting, distant metastases, and recurrence.
Associated Diseases	◘ **Meigs' Syndrome** A syndrome associated with ovarian fibroma, ascites, and pleural effusions; presents with dyspnea and pleuritic chest pain; CXR reveals pleural effusion; thoracocentesis reveals ovarian fibroma cells; ovarian US reveals tumor; treat with therapeutic thoracocentesis, diuresis; treat underlying fibroma with excision.

ID/CC	A **24-year-old** woman complains of several weeks of crampy, bilateral **lower abdominal pain worsened by menses;** thick, **greenish-yellow vaginal discharge;** and vulvar irritation. This morning she woke up with increased pain, **fever, and vomiting.**
HPI	She has had **unprotected sex** with **multiple sexual partners.** She has had an **IUD** since age 20.
PE	VS: **fever** (39 C); hypotension (BP 85/60); tachycardia (HR 110). PE: abdomen soft; hypogastric tenderness; no masses palpable; **voluntary guarding but no rigidity;** no rebound tenderness or change in bowel sounds; pelvic exam reveals **exquisite tenderness when cervix is moved** laterally (= CERVICAL MOTION TENDERNESS); **adnexa tender; abundant purulent discharge from cervical os.**
Labs	CBC: **leukocytosis** (16,000) with left shift. **Elevated ESR;** Gram stain (of purulent discharge) reveals **intracellular gram-negative diplococci** (suggestive of gonorrhea) as well as increased WBCs (18 leukocytes per HPF, suggestive of chlamydia); RPR nonreactive; blood culture shows no growth at 24 hours.
Imaging	US-Pelvis: no masses in adnexa.
Pathogenesis	Pelvic inflammatory disease (PID) refers to ascending genital infection involving the endometrium, fallopian tubes, and broad ligaments (= ENDOMETRITIS, SALPINGITIS, PARAMETRITIS). It is usually transmitted **sexually** via cervical infection with upward spread to the fallopian tubes. PID is typically a polymicrobial infection, but 60%–70% of the time *Chlamydia trachomatis* and/or *Neisseria gonorrhoeae* will infect the cervical canal, damaging the protective layer and forming adhesions and fibrosis. *Bacteroides* species, *E. coli, H. influenzae, Mycoplasma,* and, less commonly, tuberculosis (hematogenous route) may also be involved. Often the infection is polymicrobial.
Epidemiology	Incidence is highest among young females with **multiple sexual partners; unprotected sex** greatly increases the risk of developing PID. Frequent **douching,** young age, low socioeconomic status, and **smoking** are also associated with an increased risk of developing PID.

PELVIC INFLAMMATORY DISEASE

OCPs appear to have a protective effect against chlamydial PID (by thickening cervical mucus).

Management   Samples of cervical exudate (consider rectal, urethral, and throat swabs) are taken. Antibiotics are then started before results are obtained. **Ceftriaxone** 250 mg IM or **cefoxitin** 2 g IM plus 1 g **probenecid** PO followed by **doxycycline** 100 mg PO BID ×14 days is the usual outpatient regimen. For inpatients, **cefoxitin** or **cefotetan** plus **doxycycline** is used. **Clindamycin plus gentamicin** is an alternative inpatient regimen. If complications such as abscess formation or peritonitis ensue, surgical drainage may be required. Indications for hospitalization include tubo-ovarian abscess, association with an IUD, patient noncompliance, and signs of systemic infection. Refer sexual partners for treatment.

Complications   Infectivity (related to chronicity and recurrence), **infertility,** thickening of the tubal wall (= INTERSTITIAL SALPINGITIS), hydrosalpinx, peri-oophoritis, tubo-ovarian abscess formation, perforation with generalized peritonitis, dyspareunia, ectopic pregnancy, gonococcal perihepatitis (= FITZ–HUGH–CURTIS SYNDROME), intestinal obstruction due to adhesions, and suppurative arthritis.

Associated Diseases   ◻ **Adnexal Torsion** Associated with ovarian tumor or cyst; presents with abrupt, severe lower abdominal pain and mild fever; leukocytosis is often seen; laparoscopy is both diagnostic and therapeutic; complications include adnexal infarction.

◻ **Acute Pyelonephritis** Acute kidney infection, most commonly caused by *E. coli* or other Enterobacteriaceae; presents with flank pain, fever, and dysuria; UA shows WBCs and WBC casts; nitrites positive, > 105 colonies/mL on culture; treat with IV antibiotics based on sensitivities.

◻ **Appendicitis** Inflammation of the appendix secondary to lymphoid hyperplasia or fecalith obstruction; presents with epigastric pain migrating to McBurney's point in the right lower quadrant and with rebound tenderness, fever, nausea, and vomiting; treat with appendectomy; complications include perforation, peritonitis, and sepsis.

◼ **Ectopic Pregnancy** Gestation in a location other than the endometrium, usually in the ampulla of the fallopian tube; risk factors include previous tubal surgery, endometriosis, IUD use, and PID; presents with amenorrhea, pelvic pain, vaginal spotting, and cervical tenderness; hCG levels lower than expected; US shows no products of conception in the uterine cavity; treat by laparoscopic linear salpingostomy, segmental resection, or methotrexate.

ID/CC	A **20-year-old** woman complains **of inability to conceive, excessive menstrual flow, and bilateral lower abdominal pain.**
HPI	She was treated for **pulmonary tuberculosis** a few years ago and has been unable to conceive for the past two years. Semen analysis of her husband is normal.
PE	VS: normal HR; normal BP; low-grade fever. PE: **small, fixed adnexal masses** that are **matted and fixed to uterus** (= "FROZEN PELVIS"); uterine tenderness; thickening of broad ligament.
Labs	CBC: anemia. **Elevated ESR;** culture of endometrial curettage reveals *Mycobacterium tuberculosis;* histologic examination of curettage shows presence of characteristic **tubercles; Mantoux test strongly positive;** ELISA for TB positive.
Imaging	XR-Chest: **fibrotic shadows** (old healed pulmonary tuberculosis). Hysterosalpingography (HSG) is contraindicated in a proven case of tuberculosis.
Pathogenesis	Pelvic tuberculosis usually occurs when a primary lung infection invades the pelvis hematogenously. The **fallopian tube** is the most frequently involved part of the genital tract.
Epidemiology	Incidence peaks in early 20s. May follow IUD insertion, hysterosalpingography, and D&C.
Management	**Four-drug therapy** with INH, pyrazinamide, ethambutol, and rifampin for two months; continue INH and rifampin for another six months. **Indications for surgery** include disease progression or persistence despite chemotherapy; **90% of cases are cured** with chemotherapy, but **only 10% regain fertility.**
Complications	Complications include INH-induced **pyridoxine deficiency** (administer pyridoxine) and **hepatotoxicity** resulting from rifampin and INH (obtain baseline LFTs). **Adhesions** within the uterine cavity form synechiae (= ASHERMAN'S SYNDROME).
Associated Diseases	◘ **Actinomycosis** Infection by *Actinomyces israelii;* presents with abscess of the neck/jaw, abdomen, or chest; causes classic draining sinuses with "sulfur granules"; the disease readily crosses tissue planes and

invades bone; biopsy or smear shows branching hyphae-like bacteria; treat with penicillin.

ID/CC	A **23-year-old obese** female complains of **facial hair** (= HIRSUTISM) that she shaves several times a week.
HPI	She also complains of intermittent **lower abdominal pain** and **heaviness** off and on as well as **lack of menstruation** for the past six months (= SECONDARY AMENORRHEA). (Patients may also show increased bleeding due to endometrial hyperplasia from unopposed estrogenic stimulation.) For the past three years, she has been trying to become pregnant (= INFERTILITY).
PE	VS: normal. PE: **obese;** increased hair on face, back, and arms; acne and frontal balding; normal breast development; no clitoromegaly; external genitalia normal; **ovaries enlarged** bilaterally.
Labs	**Elevated LH;** low FSH; **increased LH to FSH ratio (> 3:1);** normal prolactin; **increased free testosterone, DHEA, and androstenedione;** increased ratio of estrone to estradiol; hyperglycemia.
Imaging	US: **multiple ovarian cysts** bilaterally.
Pathogenesis	Idiopathic etiology and associated with family history; also known as **Stein–Leventhal syndrome.** It is characterized by **anovulatory cycles** (with loss of midcycle temperature elevation), **excess ovarian androgen** production, and multiple ovarian cysts. Obesity is common; androstenedione undergoes aromatization to estrone in fat tissue. Estrone stimulates LH and suppresses FSH secretion, which further leads to the vicious cycle of LH causing increased androgen production.
Epidemiology	Polycystic ovarian disease (PCOD) is the **most common cause of hirsutism** and is usually seen in females in their **late teens and young adulthood;** rarely it is associated with prior CNS injury and hyperprolactinemia. PCOD increases the risk of developing type 2 diabetes.
Management	Rule out other possible causes of anovulation and hirsutism (e.g., thyroid disease, androgen-secreting tumors); **weight loss** results in symptomatic improvement in many patients as well as return of menses and ovulation. Estrone-positive feedback on the pituitary must be broken if the disease is to be treated correctly. **OCPs** increase steroid hormone–binding

POLYCYSTIC OVARIAN DISEASE

globulin and suppress the increased LH production with a consequent decrease in free testosterone and androstenedione and the return of a regular, albeit artificial, menstruation. **Induction of ovulation** by clomiphene may be attempted. **Cyproterone acetate** is still an experimental progestational agent and antiandrogen that is useful in the management of hirsutism.

Complications   Endometrial hyperplasia and carcinoma; multiple pregnancy after clomiphene-induced ovulation.

Associated Diseases   N/A

ID/CC	A **34-year-old** female complains of **breast pain** that is partially relieved by OTC analgesics, together with **depression, anxiety,** and a loss of interest in pleasurable activities (= ANHEDONIA) just prior to **the onset of her periods.**
HPI	The patient also feels "swollen" and **irritable** and often has **headaches** during this time. With the onset of menses these complaints disappear, but **colicky lower abdominal pain** occurs, sometimes incapacitating her (= DYSMENORRHEA). She is a **smoker,** has irritable bowel syndrome, and was previously admitted for paroxysmal supraventricular tachycardia. She suffered **postpartum depression** following the birth of her two children.
PE	VS: **tachycardia** (HR 110); mild hypotension (BP 100/60); mild tachypnea (RR 24); no fever. PE: well hydrated and **anxious-appearing.**
Labs	CBC/UA: normal. Lytes: normal (hypoglycemia has been suggested in pathogenesis). TFTs and cortisol normal (to rule out hypo- or hyperthyroidism as well as hypopituitarism or Addison's).
Imaging	CXR/KUB: normal. US-Abdomen: no apparent pathology.
Pathogenesis	Premenstrual tension syndrome (PMTS) is not fully understood and has a **multifactorial** pathogenesis involving psychiatric, physiologic, and endocrine factors such as estrogen-progesterone imbalance, hyperprolactinemia, hyperaldosteronism, and hypoglycemia. In the diagnosis of PMTS, the **relationship of the symptoms to the menstrual period** is more important than the nature of the symptoms, since a wide constellation of symptoms are included in the syndrome. Key to the diagnosis of PMTS is the presence of a **"disease-free period" during the follicular phase** of the cycle.
Epidemiology	PMTS is seen with increasing frequency in patients with **preexisting depression** and those who suffered from **postpartum depression.** There is also a higher incidence in the fourth and fifth decades. Patients with PMTS may also have illnesses such as gastritis, colitis, migraine,

21.   **PREMENSTRUAL TENSION SYNDROME**

asthma, allergies, and neurodermatitis.

Management	The diagnosis is one of exclusion; major causes of organic disease must be ruled out with appropriate lab tests, psychiatric evaluation, endoscopy, and pelvic ultrasound. **Exercise,** a high-protein diet, and pyridoxine, vitamin E, and magnesium supplements may improve symptoms. **OCPs, NSAIDs,** diuretics, medroxyprogesterone, and fluoxetine may be effective if other therapies have failed. **Counseling** or referral to a mental health professional is often appropriate.
Complications	Chronicity, failure of medical treatment, and periodic disability.
Associated Diseases	N/A

. . . .

21. PREMENSTRUAL TENSION SYNDROME

ID/CC	A 20-year-old woman presents for an evaluation of **amenorrhea.**
HPI	She has **never menstruated.** She complains of **swelling in the inguinal region.**
PE	**Tall** with **eunuchoid features; breasts large** but with sparse glandular tissue; nipples and areolae pale; **no axillary or pubic hair; bilateral inguinal hernias (ectopic testes);** labia minora underdeveloped; vagina ends as **blind sac.**
Labs	Karyotype: **46, XY.** Serum **testosterone levels normal for male;** biopsy of removed testes reveals **no evidence of spermatogenesis.**
Imaging	US: **absent uterus and rudimentary fallopian tubes;** no ovaries.
Pathogenesis	Testicular feminization is inherited as an **X-linked recessive trait** resulting in the **absence of testosterone receptors;** individuals have a 46, XY genotype and a female phenotype. Because müllerian inhibiting factor is secreted, these individuals have an absence of müllerian-derived structures.
Epidemiology	The incidence of primary amenorrhea is < 3%, with testicular feminization accounting for 10% of all cases.
Management	Patients are usually regarded socially as **female; gonadectomy** is performed because of the increased risk (50%) **of testicular neoplasia.** Estrogen treatment is given for maintaining secondary sexual characteristics. Surgical treatment involves creation of a vagina.
Complications	Confused gender identity and infertility.
Associated Diseases	◻ **Klinefelter's Syndrome** Also known as testicular dysgenesis; the most common cause of male hypogonadism; presents with increased height, eunuchoid body habitus, gynecomastia, testicular atrophy, and impotence; karyotype 47, XXY; treat with androgen replacement.

ID/CC	A 17-year-old girl is brought by her mother to a gynecologist because her **periods have not yet begun** (= PRIMARY AMENORRHEA).
HPI	She underwent surgical repair for **coarctation of the aorta** a few years ago.
PE	VS: normal. PE: **short in stature; low-set ears;** breasts, pubic and axillary hair, and external genitalia not developed; **short, webbed neck; shield chest** with widely spaced nipples; increased **carrying angle at elbow** (= CUBITUS VALGUS).
Labs	**Low estradiol;** high pituitary gonadotropins. Karyotype: **45, XO** (consistent with diagnosis of Turner's syndrome).
Imaging	US: "streak" dysgenetic ovaries.
Pathogenesis	Most patients with Turner's syndrome have a **45, XO karyotype;** others have an alteration in the structure of one of the X chromosomes or exhibit a **mosaic pattern** for two or more cell lines (usually 45, X and either 46, XY or 46, XX). A mosaic pattern will result in various degrees of **gonadal dysgenesis, secondary amenorrhea, and premature menopause;** if a Y chromosome is present in the genotype, the risk of **gonadoblastomas** makes gonadectomy advisable.
Epidemiology	Incidence is 1 in 2,500–10,000 live female births.
Management	**Estrogen replacement therapy.** If diagnosis is made in childhood, short stature can be treated with **oxandrolone and/or growth hormone.** Cyclical use of estrogen and progesterone will initiate regular menstrual bleeding although infertility persists.
Complications	Gonadal neoplasia and infertility.
Associated Diseases	N/A

PRIMARY AMENORRHEA - TURNER'S SYNDROME

ID/CC	A **17-year-old** female seeks a gynecologic consultation for **cessation of menses** (= SECONDARY AMENORRHEA).
HPI	She was admitted to the hospital in an **emaciated** state and was diagnosed with anorexia nervosa. Her parents report that she has experienced **marked weight loss** (about 18 kg) over the past two years. Her menarche was at age 14.
PE	VS: orthostatic hypotension; hypothermia (36.5 C); bradycardia. PE: emaciated; weight below 10th percentile for age and height; secondary sexual characteristics developed; no signs of pregnancy; peripheral edema (due to hypoalbuminemia).
Labs	CBC: anemia; leukopenia; relative lymphocytosis; thrombocytopenia. Urine pregnancy test negative; **estrogen levels markedly suppressed; gonadotropin levels low;** low ESR; hypercholesterolemia; elevated BUN; decreased LH and FSH; low T4 and T3.
Imaging	N/A
Pathogenesis	**Inability to maintain 85% of ideal weight.** Although **hypothalamic dysfunction** is postulated to be the most likely mechanism, the disease is multifactorial.
Epidemiology	Occurs in up to 1% of females aged 12–18.
Management	**Weight gain** often restores the hypothalamic-pituitary-ovarian axis; **hormone replacement therapy** is instituted as prophylaxis against osteoporosis. **Referral to specialists** or **hospitalization** may be indicated (often for underlying psychiatric disorders).
Complications	Malnutrition, electrolyte disturbances, dehydration, vitamin deficiency, and cardiovascular collapse.
Associated Diseases	N/A

SECONDARY AMENORRHEA -
ANOREXIA NERVOSA

ID/CC	A 35-year-old woman complains of **galactorrhea, visual field defects, and inability to conceive.**
HPI	The patient has been **amenorrheic** for the past six months (= SECONDARY AMENORRHEA) and also feels that her **field of vision** is **constricted;** she denies use of any medications or drugs. She has a healthy 7-year-old son (secondary infertility), is not using any contraceptives, and wishes to conceive.
PE	Visual field charting reveals **bitemporal hemianopia;** pelvic exam unremarkable; **breasts express milk** readily on pressure.
Labs	Pregnancy test negative; **TSH normal; elevated prolactin** (> 2500 mU/L) (suggestive of macroadenoma); breast biopsy normal.
Imaging	**[A]** CT: enhancing **pituitary macroadenoma** (> 10 mm) **compressing the optic chiasm. [B]** CT-Coronal: another case with an enhancing pituitary fossa mass.
Pathogenesis	Hyperprolactinemia is defined as a prolactin level of > 800 mU/L and is considered significant when accompanied by oligomenorrhea. Hyperprolactinemia interferes with the menstrual cycle by suppressing the pulsatility of LH release from the pituitary; common causes include **prolactin-producing tumors, primary hypothyroidism, drugs** such as metoclopramide and phenothiazines, and **chronic renal failure.** It may also be **idiopathic.**
Epidemiology	Prolactinomas are present in > 10% of the population.
Management	**Bromocriptine** followed by **surgical** resection; **fertility is usually restored** after treatment. For tumors < 10 mm, bromocriptine with annual CT/MR. If menses do not resume, ovulation induction may be achieved with clomiphene citrate.
Complications	Infertility and panhypopituitarism.
Associated Diseases	N/A

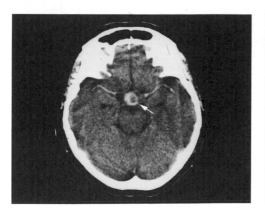 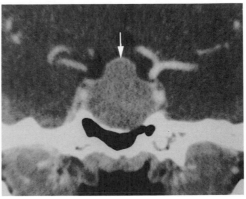

SECONDARY AMENORRHEA –
PROLACTINOMA

ID/CC	A 35-year-old woman presents with confusion, **abrupt-onset high fever, vomiting, diarrhea,** and **severe headache.**
HPI	She developed an extensive **skin rash** two days ago followed by a **high-grade fever and chills** today. Her husband says she uses a **diaphragm for contraception.**
PE	VS: **tachycardia** (HR 110); **fever** (39.2 C); **hypotension** (< 90 mm systolic). PE: toxic-appearing; drowsy but responding to verbal commands; **scarlatiniform rash** seen over entire body; **pharyngeal, conjunctival, and vaginal mucosae congested;** no neck rigidity or Kernig's sign; fundus normal; no localizing neurologic deficit found.
Labs	CBC: **leukocytosis; anemia; thrombocytopenia** (< 100,000). UA: mild pyuria. BUN and creatinine elevated; **CPK elevated.** LFTs: **elevated bilirubin; elevated AST and ALT.** Blood culture negative (illness due to toxin, not invasion of the organism); vaginal cultures yield *S. aureus.* LP: CSF normal.
Imaging	N/A
Pathogenesis	Result of localized staphylococcal soft-tissue infections arising from tumors, abscesses and abrasions, burns, osteomyelitis, and postsurgical infection. The effects of the disease are mediated through the **exotoxin TSST-1,** which functions as a **superantigen,** stimulating the production of **interleukin-1** and **tumor necrosis factor** and the release of endotoxin. **Superabsorbent tampons** obstruct menstrual outflow, causing retrograde flow and peritoneal seeding with bacteria.
Epidemiology	Staphylococcal toxic shock syndrome (TSS) has been associated with the use of **vaginal contraceptive sponges and tampons. Most cases of TSS occur in menstruating women.** With the elimination of suspect superabsorbent tampons and more judicious use of ordinary tampons, the incidence of staphylococcal TSS associated with menstruation has declined; nonmenstrual cases now account for > 20% of current cases. Most patients recover in 1–2 weeks; the mortality rate is approximately 5%.
Management	Immediate treatment of **hypotension and shock** with

vigorous fluid replacement (and supplemental catecholamines if needed), drainage of any staphylococcal abscesses, and **systemic antimicrobial therapy** with a beta-lactamase-resistant penicillin or a cephalosporin.

Complications   Up to 30% of women may have recurrences.

Associated Diseases   ◘ **Rocky Mountain Spotted Fever** Caused by *Rickettsia rickettsii;* vector is wood tick; presents with a peripheral petechial rash on the palms and soles; positive Weil–Felix reaction; treat with chloramphenicol and tetracyclines.

ID/CC A 35-year-old female complains of **intense vaginal itching and discomfort.**

HPI She also complains of a **malodorous, profuse, frothy gray discharge.** She is not using any barrier contraceptives.

PE VS: normal HR and BP; no fever. PE: cervix and vaginal mucosa appear visibly irritated and inflamed; **"strawberry spots"** on vaginal wall and cervix; malodorous, frothy gray discharge confirmed.

Labs **Vaginal pH > 4.5;** saline smear reveals **presence of motile trichomonads** and PMNs (diagnostic even if only one trichomonad is seen); KOH smear unremarkable.

Imaging N/A

Pathogenesis Caused by the **sexually transmitted *Trichomonas vaginalis;*** semen, menstrual blood, or processes that alter vaginal pH increase susceptibility to infection. *Trichomonas* may also be seen on Pap smear.

Epidemiology *Trichomonas* vaginitis is as common as gonorrhea among sexually active women.

Management Treat both patient and partner with a 2-g single dose of **metronidazole.** Vinegar douching decreases parasite load and markedly reduces symptoms.

Complications Complications include cervical and vaginal epithelial changes resulting in false-positive Pap smears. Patients taking metronidazole should not drink alcohol, as it leads to a **disulfiram-like reaction.**

Associated Diseases ◘ **Bacterial Vaginosis** *Gardnerella vaginalis* is the most common etiology; may occur with other anaerobes; presents with a malodorous discharge and vaginal irritation; increased vaginal pH (> 4.5); discharge has positive "whiff" test on KOH prep, "clue" cells on microscopy; treat with metronidazole.

◘ **Candidal Vaginitis** The most common cause of vaginitis; risk increases with immunodeficiency, antibiotic or oral contraceptive use, pregnancy, and diabetes; presents with vaginal irritation, dysuria, and characteristic "cottage-cheese" discharge; budding yeast, hyphae, and pseudohyphae on KOH prep; treat with

27. TRICHOMONAS VAGINITIS

topical antifungal agents (e.g., clotrimazole) or oral fluconazole.

ID/CC	A 43-year-old **black** female complains of **frequent, profuse, nonpainful menstrual periods** (bleeding is the most common presenting symptom of uterine leiomyomata).
HPI	The patient has been having **urinary frequency** (due to pressure on the bladder) without any pain or hematuria. She is mildly hypertensive, is on beta-blockers and diuretics, and has not seen a doctor for five years.
PE	VS: normal. PE: no gum or subcutaneous bleeding; mild pallor; **irregular, mobile, nontender, firm pelvic mass; enlarged and irregular uterus** with multiple firm and round **nodularities** on anterior and posterior aspects; adnexa nonpalpable; no leg edema.
Labs	CBC/PBS: **hypochromic, microcytic anemia** (chronic iron deficiency anemia due to increased bleeding). Normal ESR. Lytes/UA: normal. TFTs, PT/PTT, and INR normal.
Imaging	**[A]** US-Pelvis: a large, round, hypoechoic mass is seen on the uterus. **[B]** US-Pelvis: two discrete hypoechoic areas are seen in the uterus in another patient. **[C]** XR-Pelvis: calcification of a fibroid is demonstrated in another patient.
Pathogenesis	Leiomyomas (= UTERINE FIBROIDS) are benign, **estrogen-dependent** tumors of unknown etiology consisting of myometrium. They may be **subserosal** (on the serosal side of the uterine wall), **intramural** (located in the myometrium; most common type), or **submucosal** (protruding toward the uterine cavity). Submucosal leiomyomas are most likely to cause irregular bleeding (due to distortion of the endometrium and blood supply).
Epidemiology	Fibroids are the **most common tumors affecting women** and the most common surgical indication for hysterectomy. They have a higher incidence in blacks and occur more frequently in the later premenopausal years; after menopause, they tend to atrophy and calcify.
Management	**Endometrial malignancy or hyperplasia** must be ruled out by endometrial biopsy in patients who present with bleeding during the late premenopausal or early postmenopausal period. A **Pap smear** is also indicated to

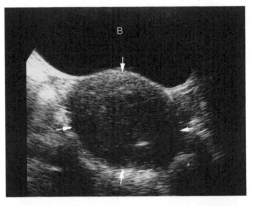

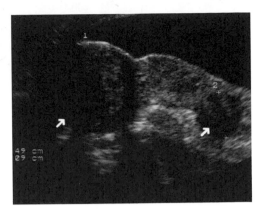

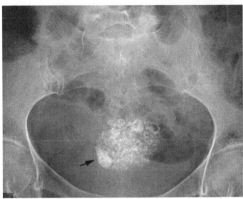

rule out cervical cancer. Many cases may be managed by close observation with frequent follow-up to prevent anemia and detect tumor growth. In some patients, large leiomyomata impinging on the uterine cavity cause infertility or recurrent abortions, in which case a **myomectomy** is warranted. If a patient is symptomatic but perimenopausal, a conservative approach may be used consisting of **cyclical progestogens** or GnRH antagonists until the onset of menopause. **Hysterectomy** is the procedure of choice for symptomatic females who have completed childbirth.

Complications　Complications include profuse **hemorrhage; pelvic pain** due to twisting of mass or infarction; **infertility;** malignant transformation (rare); hydronephrosis due to mass effect and pressure on ureters; protrusion of large submucous myomas with risk of infection; and calcific, hyaline (most common), or hemorrhagic degeneration. During pregnancy there is also an increased incidence of spontaneous abortions, postpartum bleeding, and breech presentations.

Associated Diseases　▪ **Endometrial Carcinoma** The most common gynecologic malignancy; associated with unopposed estrogen exposure; commonly presents with postmenopausal vaginal bleeding; diagnosed with Pap smear, endocervical curettage, and endometrial biopsy; treat with TAH-BSO followed by radiation depending on the stage, adjuvant hormonal and chemotherapy for metastatic disease.

ID/CC	A 61-year-old woman complains of a **heavy sensation** in her lower abdomen made worse by straining, increased **frequency of urination,** and **burning on urination** (= DYSURIA; due to altered location of the bladder with stagnation of urine and bacterial proliferation).
HPI	She is an otherwise-healthy **multiparous female** whose children were all **delivered vaginally.** She has also experienced **leakage of urine while sneezing and coughing** (= STRESS INCONTINENCE). She has been menopausal for 12 years and has not taken hormone replacement.
PE	Inspection of external genitalia (while asking patient to bear down) reveals a mass bulging through anterior wall of vagina (= CYSTOCELE) and downward protrusion of cervix (= UTERINE PROLAPSE) (examine the patient standing so that the full extent of the protrusion can be assessed).
Labs	UA: abundant leukocytes and bacteria; alkaline pH and positive nitrates (due to infection from stagnation of urine).
Imaging	Voiding Cystourethrogram: the bladder drops below the symphysis pubis during voiding; loss of urethrovesical angle.
Pathogenesis	Childbirth causes stretching of the pelvic support structures; **increased weight** during pregnancy and the **loss of muscle tone** and estrogen that accompanies menopause exacerbate incompetence of pelvic support, resulting in cystourethrocele and uterine prolapse. Aggravating factors include obesity, chronic cough, and frequent straining. If seen in nulliparity, it is usually the result of spina bifida occulta.
Epidemiology	Most common in multiparous, postmenopausal women.
Management	Nonsurgical treatment includes avoidance of straining and lifting heavy weights, **pessary support,** topical, oral, or parenteral **estrogens,** and **pelvic floor exercises** (= KEGEL EXERCISES). **Surgery** is indicated when the patient suffers from recurrent urinary symptoms or if the cystocele is sufficiently large. If only a cystocele is present, an anterior colporrhaphy is performed; if the

29. **UTERINE PROLAPSE WITH CYSTOCELE**

degree of uterine prolapse is severe, a hysterectomy with restoration of pelvic support may be indicated.

Complications   Keratinization of the vagina, decubitus ulceration, cervical hypertrophy, obstructive lesions of the urinary tract, recurrent UTIs, and incarceration of the prolapse.

Associated Diseases   N/A

UTERINE PROLAPSE WITH CYSTOCELE

ID/CC	A **63-year-old** female complains of a thick, yellowish, **purulent discharge** and a **painful lesion** on the right vulva for two days (carcinoma is usually painless but may be painful in the presence of secondary infection).
HPI	The patient has had **vulvar pruritus** for several months, which she has been unsuccessfully treating with various creams. For the past two days, she has also noticed some bleeding and staining of her undergarments.
PE	VS: normal. PE: no abdominal masses; inguinal area reveals **rubbery, tender nodes** on affected side (due to superimposed infection); vulva shows 2.5-cm **ulcerating lesion** on posterior aspect of right labia majora with rolled, **indurated edges,** easy bleeding, signs of local infection (erythema, increase in temperature, edema, pain), and surrounding hypopigmentation; vaginal exam reveals atrophic mucosal surface; cervix normal; no pelvic masses; rectal exam reveals normal sphincter tone with no masses.
Labs	CBC: mild leukocytosis. Lytes: normal. FSH and LH elevated (due to menopause). UA: normal; urine culture and sensitivity negative. Gram stain (of exudate) reveals abundant gram-positive cocci in clusters; excisional biopsy reveals squamous cell carcinoma.
Imaging	CXR: unfolded aortic knob; mild cardiomegaly; no infiltrates; no signs of metastatic disease. IVP: normal.
Pathogenesis	**Atypical hyperplasia** and **dysplastic leukoplakia** of the vulva are considered premalignant conditions that may progress to invasive vulvar carcinoma; **human papillomavirus** (HPV 16, 18, 31, 33, 35) has been implicated in its pathogenesis. As in cervical cancer, dysplasia and carcinoma in situ precede the development of invasive carcinoma by many years. Vulvar carcinoma may be ulcerating or fungating (= EXOPHYTIC) as well as macular or papular; fungating lesions or ulcers are not always seen. The most common type is **squamous cell,** which is usually well differentiated and keratinizing. Tumors invade by local extension and by lymphatic spread. The FIGO staging system is surgical with TNM grading of the lesion as follows: **stage I** - tumor confined to the vulva/perineum (< 2 cm); **stage II** - tumor confined to the vulva/perineum (> 2 cm); **stage III** -

tumor of any size with local spread (lower urethra, vagina, or anus) or unilateral lymph node involvement; **stage IV** - widespread invasion and/or bilateral lymph node involvement.

Epidemiology	Comprises approximately 5% of all gynecologic malignancies and has an overall five-year survival rate of approximately 65%. It is usually a disease of **elderly females** with the highest incidence in the 60s.
Management	Lesions of the vulva that look premalignant should be treated by **excisional biopsy** with a margin of normal-looking tissue; several samples may be needed to detect the disease owing to its **multicentricity.** Toluidine blue and colposcopy may help guide sites for biopsy. IVP will rule out kidney/ureteral disease and will detect possible local GU invasion; sigmoidoscopy is suggested with posterior vulvar lesions. **Vulvar intraepithelial neoplasia** may be treated by skinning vulvectomy, cryosurgery, wide local excision, or laser. The verrucous type may be treated with wide local excision. **Radical vulvectomy with bilateral node dissection** is the mainstay of treatment for stages I–III. For early disease in younger patients, a more conservative approach may be tried. Radiotherapy may be used in select cases.
Complications	Local spread with infection, bleeding; vaginal and anorectal spread; lymphatic disease (incidence of about 30%; all stages; spreads to iliac, femoral, and inguinal nodes and later to deep pelvic nodes); and recurrence after surgery.
Associated Diseases	◘ **Paget's Disease of the Breast** Aggressive breast cancer with overlying skin erythema; presents with itching, burning, and discharge; superficial erosion and eczematous scaling may be apparent; biopsy shows "Paget" cells invading the dermis; requires surgical excision.
	◘ **Vulvar Leukoplakia** Disorders of the vulvar epithelium; causes include vitiligo, malignancies, dystrophies, and inflammatory processes; presents with genital discoloration and pruritus; biopsy reveals the underlying cause; treatment varies with etiology.

ID/CC	A 28-year-old primigravida at **13 weeks'** gestation complains of **vaginal passage of blood clots** with **lower abdominal pain** radiating to the back.
HPI	She had **vaginal spotting** one week ago with mild abdominal cramps. She rested for two days, after which her symptoms disappeared until the onset of her present complaints.
PE	VS: normal. PE: no acute distress; mild **hypogastric tenderness;** abdomen soft with no rigidity; no rebound tenderness; uterus soft and increased in size with an **open cervix.**
Labs	CBC/Lytes: normal. ESR normal; pregnancy test positive. UA: few RBCs.
Imaging	US: uterus increased in size; no intrauterine gestational sac.
Pathogenesis	The most common causes of first-trimester spontaneous abortion are **chromosomal abnormalities** (most commonly trisomies). In the second trimester, common causes include maternal anatomic defects such as bicornuate or septate uterus, Asherman's syndrome (intrauterine synechiae after vigorous curettage), leiomyomata, incompetent cervix, placental abnormalities, drugs (cocaine) and toxins, and maternal illnesses such as hypo/hyperthyroidism, diabetes, SLE, and infections (toxoplasmosis, HSV, listeriosis, rubella, CMV).
Epidemiology	Up to 50% of pregnancies are thought to end in spontaneous abortion (although only 15%–25% are recognized); risk factors for spontaneous abortion include **multiparity, increasing age of mother and father**, and short span between pregnancies (< 3 months). **Threatened abortion** occurs in roughly 25% of all pregnancies.
Management	Patients who have undergone abortion should be informed of **recurrence risks.** After three spontaneous abortions, **genetic counseling** is indicated. In **threatened abortion,** pelvic rest and abstinence are essential. If no fetal heart rate or gestational sac is seen on US, the fetus is evacuated. **Inevitable and incomplete abortions** are managed with D&C or vacuum suction.

ABORTION – SPONTANEOUS

For **missed abortion** up to the 28th week, prostaglandin suppositories may be used to stimulate contractions. Administration of RhoGAM (Rh immune globulin) is essential to prevent isoimmunization in subsequent pregnancies if the patient's blood type is Rh negative.

Complications Retained gestational sac–placenta fragments with persistent bleeding and infection, endometritis, parametritis, septic shock, DIC, and uterine wall perforation during D&C. **FIRST AID 2** p. 248

Associated Diseases ◘ **Dysfunctional Uterine Bleeding** Usually due to anovulation, often near menarche or menopause; presents with menstrual irregularities; treat with estrogen and progesterone.

◘ **Completed Abortion** Spontaneous passage of the entire conceptus with closure of the cervix and reduction of the uterus to normal size; presents with passage of fresh blood, blood clots, and entire conceptus via introitus; US confirms abortion; administer RhoGAM in Rh-negative women; treat by D&C and refer for psychological counseling; complications include painful cramping and hemorrhage.

◘ **Incomplete Abortion** Spontaneous passage of part of the conceptus; presents with passage of fresh blood, blood clots, and variable portions of fetal tissue via the introitus; US confirms lack of fetal heart beats and rupture of membrane; treatment is D&C to complete abortion (can wait several days to see if the abortion completes itself spontaneously); administer RhoGAM in Rh-negative women; refer for psychological counseling.

◘ **Threatened Abortion** Uterine bleeding due to any cause during the first trimester of pregnancy; presents with uterine cramping and bleeding; US detects fetal heartbeats to confirm abortion not completed; treatment is bed rest and refraining from intercourse; if abortion is inevitable (open cervical os), perform D&C; refer for psychological counseling.

◘ **Missed Abortion** Retention of dead fetus in utero for at least four weeks; presents with failure of uterine expansion on serial examinations or failure to detect fetal heart tones; US confirms the diagnosis; treatment is induction of abortion with prostaglandin or oxytocin; complications include dead fetus syndrome, which presents in the second trimester with DIC.

ID/CC	A **38-year-old** woman suddenly develops laborious breathing and lightheadedness following a vaginal delivery.
HPI	The patient is a **multigravida** (four pregnancies) who underwent complicated delivery owing to a **large fetus**. Her falling blood pressure and tachycardia were unresponsive to fluid resuscitation.
PE	VS: tachycardia (HR 110); hypotension (BP 90/60); tachypnea (RR 24). PE: **cold, clammy skin; dyspneic, cyanotic, and comatose;** weak, thready pulse; generalized tonic-clonic **convulsions** begin a few minutes afterward.
Labs	CBC: **thrombocytopenia. Decreased fibrinogen; prolonged bleeding time and PT/PTT; elevated fibrin split products** (due to DIC) and D-dimers.
Imaging	CXR: severe **pulmonary edema.**
Pathogenesis	Amniotic fluid embolism occurs when particulate matter such as hair, fetal squama-vernix, or amniotic fluid gains access to the pulmonary circulation through lacerations in the placental membrane and rupture of uterine/placental veins, producing a pulmonary embolization. Diagnosis is made on clinical grounds, since the presence of squamous cells in maternal blood is not enough to confirm a diagnosis of amniotic fluid embolism. Embolization produces severe, acute **pulmonary hypertension with hypoxemia.** The second phase gives rise to **acute heart failure and DIC a few hours afterward.**
Epidemiology	Amniotic fluid embolism is a rare complication occurring in 1 per 50,000 deliveries (after vaginal delivery, abortion, or C-section). If it occurs in the delivery period, it may be associated with **abruptio placentae** and fetal death. Predisposing factors include **older age, hypertonic labor,** use of **oxytocin,** uterine rupture, and twin pregnancy with uterine overdistention.
Management	Admission to the ICU, hemodynamic monitoring, oxygen, ventilatory support, treatment of acute heart failure, treatment of DIC.
Complications	Death in 80% of cases; neurologic damage due to

A M N I O T I C   F L U I D   E M B O L I S M

hypoxia in survivors.

Associated Diseases ◘ **Fat Embolism** Embolization of fat 24–72 hours after fracture of long bone; presents with petechiae (usually seen in the sclera), fever, dyspnea, cyanosis, and hypotension; refractory hypoxemia with hypercapnia; fat in urine and sputum; CXR with late pulmonary infiltrates; treat with ventilatory support; prevent by early stabilization of long-bone fractures.

◘ **Pulmonary Thromboembolism** Thrombus in the pulmonary artery most commonly originating from a proximal DVT; presents with fever, chest pain, acute-onset dyspnea (especially postsurgical), tachypnea, hypotension, elevated JVP, and RV gallop rhythm with widely split S2; hypoxia and hypercapnia; ECG shows sinus tachycardia; V/Q scan reveals mismatching; pulmonary angiography is the gold standard but is invasive; treat with oxygen, add tPA if the patient has fulminant hypotension, anticoagulation.

◘ **Disseminated Intravascular Coagulation** A consumptive coagulopathy characterized by excessive thrombin activity that results in fibrin deposition with thrombus formation in the microcirculation; caused by septicemia, burns, trauma, metastatic malignancy, or obstetric complications; presents with profuse bleeding (with fresh frozen plasma, platelet transfusions, cryoprecipitate, fibrinogen, or thrombotic complications); schistocytes on peripheral blood smear; low fibrinogen and platelets, prolonged PT, and elevated fibrin split products; treat the underlying cause; treat bleeding complications (with fresh frozen plasma, platelets, cryoprecipitate, fibrinogen)

ID/CC	A 26-year-old female in her **third trimester** of a twin gestation complains of **easy fatigability, weakness,** dizziness, and sleepiness for the past month.
HPI	This is the patient's second pregnancy; the first resulted in a normal full-term vaginal delivery.
PE	VS: normal. PE: **pallor;** ejection murmur I/VI in aortic area; pregnant uterus **with two fetuses,** each with normal fetal heart rate; no leg edema; normal neurologic and pelvic exams.
Labs	CBC/PBS: **low hemoglobin** with **increased MCV (=** MEGALOBLASTIC ANEMIA); leukopenia; thrombocytopenia; **hypersegmented neutrophils. Decreased reticulocyte count;** decreased serum and erythrocyte folate levels. (Normocytic, normochromic anemia is also common as a result of the dilutional effects of intravascular volume expansion.)
Imaging	US: normal development of one fetus with a slight decrease in somatometry of the second; normal amniotic fluid and placenta; no other apparent abnormalities.
Pathogenesis	In pregnancy, folate demands increase fourfold and folate absorption is decreased. **Phenytoin** and **phenobarbital** therapy, spherocytosis, hemoglobinopathies with **hemolysis, multiple gestation,** and a lack of fresh green vegetables are all predisposing factors for **megaloblastic anemia of pregnancy due to folate deficiency.** Iron deficiency is also commonly present, and a normocytic anemia may appear. The best lab test to establish the diagnosis is **RBC folate level.**
Epidemiology	The **most common cause of megaloblastic anemia in pregnancy** is **folate deficiency,** which comprises about 10% of cases of pregnancy-related anemias. It usually appears in the third trimester.
Management	Folate deficiency in pregnancy may be prevented with 1 mg of folic acid per day, which is also the **best preventive measure against** the development of **neural tube defects. Reticulocytosis** is an early sign of adequate folate replacement (also give iron if the reticulocyte count does not increase after one week).
Complications	Neural tube defects, placental abruption, and

spontaneous abortion.

Associated Diseases

◘ **Vitamin B12 Deficiency** Cofactor for DNA and myelin synthesis; deficiency is due to malabsorption (sprue, enteritis, *Diphyllobothrium latum* infection), absence of intrinsic factor (pernicious anemia), prolonged dietary deficiency (as in vegans), or terminal ileum disease; presents with anemia, degenerative changes in the spinal cord (especially the posterior columns and the corticospinal tracts), and peripheral neuropathies; hypersegmented PMNs, megaloblastic RBCs, and decreased serum vitamin B_{12}; treat the underlying disorder, IM vitamin B_{12}.

◘ **Folate Deficiency** Folate is required for DNA/RNA synthesis; deficiency is most commonly associated with alcoholism, pregnancy, or medications (Bactrim, methotrexate, phenytoin); presents with fatigue, weakness, and nausea; anemia, hypersegmented PMNs, megaloblastic RBCs, and low RBC folate; treat with folic acid supplementation; folic acid is required for patients taking Bactrim or methotrexate.

ID/CC	A 25-year-old primigravida in her early **third trimester** complains of excessive **pruritus** and **jaundice**.
HPI	The patient has been passing **dark urine** but has no history of prior jaundice, biliary colic, or dyspepsia. She is not taking any drugs and has no history of hematemesis, melena, hematochezia, or altered sensorium. She has had an uncomplicated pregnancy up to this time.
PE	VS: tachycardia (HR 105); normal BP; no fever. PE: **icterus; scratch marks** on skin; fundal height at **28 cm;** fetal parts palpable; fetal heart heard.
Labs	LFTs: **elevated serum bilirubin, predominantly conjugated; elevated alkaline phosphatase** to > 10 times normal value; **AST** and **ALT** moderately **elevated.** Serologic markers for viral hepatitis A, B, and C negative; liver biopsy reveals **intrahepatic cholestasis.**
Imaging	US-Abdomen: no evidence of cholelithiasis or choledocholithiasis; single live fetus seen.
Pathogenesis	Intrahepatic cholestasis is a hereditary metabolic defect of the liver that is usually seen in the third trimester of pregnancy; it is aggravated by high estrogen levels and is associated with OCP use. These changes resolve following delivery but recur in subsequent pregnancies.
Epidemiology	N/A
Management	Cholestyramine for control of pruritus and cholestasis; since cholestyramine interferes with the absorption of fat-soluble vitamins, **vitamin K supplementation** may be necessary. Pruritus can be treated with antihistamines. **Close prenatal and intrapartum** monitoring is necessary, and early delivery may be considered.
Complications	**Significant fetal morbidity** may result, including stillbirth, premature birth, intrapartum fetal distress, and meconium-stained amniotic fluid.
Associated Diseases	◼ **Acute Fatty Liver of Pregnancy** Unknown etiology; occurs in the third trimester; presents with abdominal pain, jaundice, nausea, and vomiting; elevated PT/PTT, bilirubin, and transaminases; requires immediate delivery; complications include hepatic encephalopathy.

34.   **CHOLESTATIC JAUNDICE OF PREGNANCY**

ID/CC	A 33-year-old woman in her **36th week of pregnancy** complains of new-onset **abdominal pain with fever and chills.**
HPI	She is a **smoker** with no medical history. She reports that "**some water**" **ran down her thighs 24 hours ago** (smoking increases incidence of premature rupture of membranes, or PROM).
PE	VS: **fever** (39.5 C); **tachycardia** (HR 110); normal BP. PE: in acute distress; **uterine tenderness;** thick, yellowish-green **cervical discharge;** cervical dilatation 3 cm; cul-de-sac **fluid nitrazine positive** (amniotic fluid, alkaline pH); **positive ferning** (sodium chloride in amniotic fluid crystallizes); **fetal tachycardia** (HR 160) with loss of variability and no decelerations.
Labs	CBC: anemia; leukocytosis (16,000) with neutrophilia. UA/Lytes: normal. TFTs normal.
Imaging	US: **scant amniotic fluid** (due to PROM); no fetal abnormalities except for tachycardia.
Pathogenesis	Chorioamnionitis, or **infection of the fetal membrane,** is most frequently caused by ascending infections and hematogenous spread. The most common causative organisms are **group B streptococcus, anaerobic streptococci,** *E. coli,* **and** *Bacteroides.* Risk factors include nulliparity, PROM, prolonged labor, ruptured membranes, preexisting infections, and multiple digital vaginal examinations.
Epidomiology	Chorioamnionitis complicates about 1% of all deliveries. In PROM of > 18 hours, there is a significantly higher incidence of chorioamnionitis; in preterm PROM the incidence may reach 25%.
Management	**Antibiotic therapy** includes ampicillin, gentamicin, and clindamycin. Antibiotics are adjusted according to culture results. Delivery may be indicated based on fetal lung maturity.
Complications	Failure to progress, C-section, endometritis (signs of infection that persist longer than 24 hours after delivery), myometritis, parametritis, septicemia, DIC, renal shutdown, and ARDS.
Associated Diseases	N/A

35. **CHORIOAMNIONITIS**

ID/CC	A 40-year-old woman presents with increasing **shortness of breath** (= DYSPNEA) and **blood-tinged sputum** (= HEMOPTYSIS; due to pulmonary metastases); she also complains of severe **nausea,** occasional vomiting, and **intermittent vaginal bleeding.**
HPI	The patient had a D&C six months ago for a **hydatidiform mole.**
PE	VS: normal. PE: **pallor;** scattered rales in lungs; no abdominal masses; **increase in size of uterus;** no adnexal masses; speculum exam reveals **bluish-red vascular tumor.**
Labs	CBC: mild anemia. LFTs: alkaline phosphatase normal. TFTs normal. UA: normal. **Elevated serum and urinary hCG** levels.
Imaging	CXR: multiple nodules (= CANNONBALL METASTASES). US-Pelvis: increased size of uterus, with solid echogenic material in the myometrium compatible with choriocarcinoma.
Pathogenesis	Choriocarcinoma is a **highly anaplastic gestational trophoblastic malignancy** (the spectrum of the disease also includes hydatidiform mole and invasive mole) that involves the proliferation of trophoblast cells but does not contain villi. It may develop during or after any pregnancy (normal or abnormal). Levels of hCG should return to normal by 12 weeks after molar pregnancy evacuation; if the level plateaus or rises or if it increases in the absence of pregnancy after having returned to normal, choriocarcinoma should be strongly suspected. It invades locally and disseminates early hematogenously; the **most common sites of spread are the lungs and vagina.** Sometimes the first signs of choriocarcinoma are metastases to the external genitalia, vagina, or rectum. Stage patients according to FIGO as follows: I = confined to the uterus; II = vaginal or pelvic metastases; III = lung metastases; and IV = other distant metastases.
Epidemiology	Most commonly develops after evacuation of a hydatidiform mole, although only 10% of complete molar pregnancies degenerate into malignancy. Factors associated with poor prognosis are hCG levels > 40,000; disease of > 4 months' duration; brain/liver metastases; failure of prior chemotherapy; and antecedent term

pregnancy.

Management Chemotherapy may consist of methotrexate or actinomycin D alone (in nonmetastatic disease or in metastatic disease with a good prognosis) or triple therapy with chlorambucil, actinomycin D, and methotrexate (in metastatic disease with a poor prognosis). Radiotherapy may be employed in disease involving brain or liver metastases.

Complications Complications include CNS, liver, and kidney metastases; bone marrow aplasia with pancytopenia due to chemotherapy; oral and GI ulcers; and elevated liver enzymes. Beta-hCG has partial TSH activity, which may cause thyrotoxicosis.

Associated Diseases ◘ **Hydatidiform Mole** Results from the fertilization of an empty ovum by normal sperm; presents with first-trimester bleeding, passage of vesicles per vagina, or hyperemesis; first-trimester preeclampsia (hypertension, edema, and proteinuria) is characteristic; beta-hCG markedly elevated; typical "snowstorm" pattern on pelvic US; requires immediate evacuation of uterine contents; complications include development of an invasive mole or choriocarcinoma.

ID/CC	A 4-month-old male is brought to a physician with a **bluish rash on his face and trunk.**
HPI	The child has had yellowing of the eyes and failure to gain weight. In addition, he has been **behaving as though he were deaf.** There is a history of a **maternal rash** (maculopapular) **during the first trimester.** The mother did not receive prenatal care.
PE	Growth retardation; **microcephaly** and bulging anterior fontanelle; **icterus; "blueberry muffin" skin lesions; microphthalmia with cataract** of left eye; discrete **black patchy pigmentation in retina; hepatosplenomegaly;** continuous cardiac **"machinery murmur."**
Labs	LFTs: increased direct and indirect serum bilirubin. **Rubella virus isolated** from urine and saliva; **IgM-specific rubella antibody positive;** bilateral **sensorineural deafness.**
Imaging	XR-Bones: metaphyseal lucent bands and trabecular irregularity extending longitudinally from the epiphysis **("celery-stalk" appearance).** Echo (with doppler): **PDA.**
Pathogenesis	Rubella virus is an **RNA togavirus** that crosses the placenta. Congenital rubella syndrome has a multi-organ manifestation in which cardiac malformations (PDA, intra-VSD, pulmonary artery stenosis), ocular lesions (cataracts, microphthalmos, chorioretinitis), and CNS abnormalities (mental retardation, microcephaly, deafness) are common. Malformation of bone metaphyses may also be present with hepatosplenomegaly, thrombocytopenia, thrombocytopenic purpura, interstitial pneumonitis, and myocarditis. **Congenitally affected infants may shed virus for several months and need to be isolated until viral cultures are negative.**
Epidemiology	Fetal abnormalities are **most likely to occur if maternal infection is within the first two months of gestation.** Immune status testing should be performed for women of childbearing age and for hospital employees who have no history of rubella vaccination. Individuals who are seronegative **should be vaccinated when not pregnant.**
Management	No specific antiviral therapy is available; appropriate treatment for specific defects is recommended. Vaccinate

CONGENITAL RUBELLA

immediately postpartum. Contraception should be used for three months after vaccination in light of the risk of fetal transmission.

Complications See Pathogenesis.

Associated Diseases ◘ **Congenital Toxoplasmosis** Transplacental transmission; primary infection is derived from consumption of raw meat or contact with cat feces; presents with neonatal hydrocephalus, retardation, and seizures; MR or CT reveals intracranial ring-enhancing, calcified lesions; treat with pyrimethamine and sulfadiazine; avoid exposure.

◘ **HIV Transmission in Pregnancy** Vertical transmission of HIV most commonly occurring in the third trimester or during birth; presents with acute retroviral syndrome (e.g., fever, malaise, adenopathy) in the first months of life; PCR detection of HIV from newborn's blood; prevention is the treatment; give AZT to the mother during the third trimester or at least during labor, markedly diminishing the rate of transmission (from 24% to 8%).

◘ **Syphilis – Congenital** Intrapartum transmission; presents with a maculopapular skin rash, mucopurulent rhinitis, peg-shaped central incisors (= HUTCHINSON'S TEETH), deafness, and osteitis; VDRL positive; treat with penicillin.

ID/CC	A 35-year-old pregnant woman is admitted because of a **complicated obstetric history with gestational diabetes.**
HPI	The patient is at 10 weeks' gestation. **During her first pregnancy she had gestational diabetes** and was prescribed insulin; her first pregnancy resulted in sudden unexpected fetal death at 36 weeks. Her second pregnancy resulted in a term **macrosomic infant weighing 4,500 g following a difficult vaginal delivery;** the baby suffered intraventricular hemorrhage and died shortly after birth. During both pregnancies, the patient had **irregular prenatal care** and **did not adhere to her insulin schedule.** Her **father is diabetic.**
PE	VS: normal. PE: **obese;** pelvic exam reveals 10-week uterus; fetal heart heard on doppler.
Labs	Fasting blood **glucose 160 mg/dL** (if value is < 140 mg/dL, retest at 24–28 weeks; if value is > 140 mg/dL, proceed to glucose tolerance test). UA: **glucosuria. Glucose tolerance test is consistent with gestational diabetes.** (In the three-hour glucose tolerance test, 100 g of glucose is administered orally and serial blood glucose levels are checked at fasting, one-, two, and three-hour intervals. The following are considered **abnormally high values: fasting > 105 mg/dL; 1 hr > 190 mg/dL; 2 hr > 165 mg/dL; 3 hr > 145 mg/dL.** If the patient has abnormal glucose levels at any two of these four time points, gestational diabetes is diagnosed.)
Imaging	US-Pelvis: single, intrauterine fetus at 10 weeks with evidence of fetal heart activity.
Pathogenesis	Caused by insulin resistance during pregnancy that is thought to be due to placental lactogen (which blocks insulin receptors) and elevated circulating estrogen and progesterone.
Epidemiology	Gestational diabetes must be suspected in all women with **significant glucosuria** on two occasions prenatally or in a single fasting urine sample; with a family history of diabetes; with previous babies weighing > 90th percentile for gestational age and sex; or with a history of previous unexpected perinatal death, polyhydramnios, or maternal obesity. **Routine prenatal screening is recommended at 24–28 weeks for all women and at**

initial visit for women who are at increased risk (see predisposing factors above). Women with gestational diabetes are at increased risk of developing diabetes in the future.

Management	Prescribe the ADA diet; institute **insulin therapy with strict blood glucose monitoring** when necessary. Oral hypoglycemics are contraindicated during pregnancy because they cross the placenta and produce fetal hypoglycemia. Perform regular prenatal checkups and tests (including glucose profiles, urinalysis, and glycosylated hemoglobin), and use US to screen the fetus for malformations.
Complications	**Maternal risks** include **retinopathy, nephropathy, neuropathy** and increased risk of **polyhydramnios, preeclampsia,** and **UTIs. Fetal risks** include **congenital malformations** (cardiac and craniospinal defects); **sacral agenesis** (a rare anomaly specifically associated with diabetes); **sudden unexpected fetal death** during the last 4–6 weeks of pregnancy; difficult delivery (shoulder dystocia) due to **macrosomia;** and neonatal problems such as **birth trauma, hyaline membrane disease, hypoglycemia,** hypomagnesemia, **hypocalcemia,** and **jaundice.** All risks are increased by poor glycemic control, especially if ketoacidosis develops.
Associated Diseases	N/A

ID/CC	A 20-year-old female complains of **nausea**, especially in the morning, and **fatigue**.
HPI	Her **last menstrual period was 10 weeks ago**, and she had repeated unprotected intercourse approximately three months ago. Her menstrual periods have been regular with average flow and no dysmenorrhea. She has also noted **increased frequency of micturition** (due to an increase in GFR).
PE	VS: normal. PE: **breasts full and tender;** pelvic exam reveals a **soft cervix** (= GOODELL'S SIGN) that is **congested and cyanotic** (= CHADWICK'S SIGN); on bimanual examination, cervix and uterine body feel like two separate organs (due to **marked softening of the isthmus**) (= HEGAR'S SIGN); uterus enlarged to 10–12 weeks' size.
Labs	**Urine pregnancy test (hCG agglutination inhibition) positive.** (Quantitative hCG assays in maternal blood are extremely sensitive and may confirm pregnancy in patients where the diagnosis is uncertain.)
Imaging	**[A]** US-Pelvis: another case in which a six-week gestation is demonstrated. **[B]** US-Abdomen: a gestation of 16 weeks is shown in another patient; note the abdomen (1) and head (2).
Pathogenesis	N/A
Epidemiology	N/A
Management	Inform the patient of the pregnancy and give appropriate advice regarding **drugs** (to prevent teratogenic insult), **nutrition** (a balanced diet and supplementation with iron and folic acid), **exercise** (moderate exercise along with avoidance of strenuous work), **travel** (avoidance of long-distance travel before 12 weeks and after 28 weeks), and **regular prenatal care** (monthly intervals until 28 weeks, then every 3 weeks until 32 weeks, every 2 weeks until 36 weeks, and every week thereafter). At the initial prenatal visit, the following labs should be ordered: CBC, blood grouping and cross-matching, rubella antibody titer, cervical gonorrhea and chlamydia cultures, VDRL, HBsAg, Pap smear, UA for glucose, protein, and microscopic exam, PPD, blood glucose, and ELISA for HIV. Standard procedures that are routinely

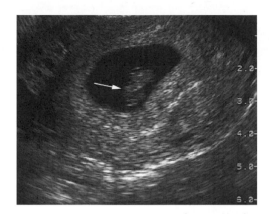 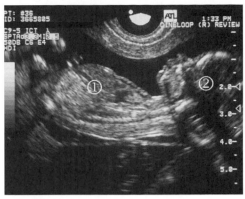

performed after the initial visit include the following: **before 12 weeks:** transvaginal ultrasound is the most accurate means of estimating gestational age (intrauterine gestational sac with a fetal pole and positive heartbeat can be identified as early as six weeks of gestation). At **15–20 weeks:** triple screen as follows: (1) maternal serum alpha-fetoprotein (AFP); (2) hCG; and (3) unconjugated estriol to identify neural tube defects (elevated AFP, low hCG, and elevated estriol), trisomy 21 (low AFP, elevated hCG, and low estriol), or trisomy 18 (low AFP, low hCG, and low estriol). At **18–20 weeks:** US to assess fetal development. At **24–28 weeks:** glucose tolerance test (one at initial visit if risk factors are present). At **28–30 weeks:** RhoGAM administered to Rh-negative patients. At **34–38 weeks:** CBC repeated. At **36–40 weeks:** cervical chlamydia, gonorrhea, and group B streptococcus cultures in high-risk patients.

Complications   N/A

Associated Diseases   N/A

ID/CC	A 29-year-old G1P0 at 37 weeks' gestation presents with severe **headache, visual impairment,** and dull **right upper quadrant abdominal pain** of four hours' duration; while in the ambulance, she had a generalized tonic-clonic **seizure.**
HPI	She is an otherwise-healthy **Hispanic** immigrant of **low socioeconomic status** and is in the ninth month of her **first pregnancy** (primigravida); two months ago her family practitioner treated her for **hand and face edema, high blood pressure, and proteinuria** (= PREECLAMPSIA). Over the past three weeks she has noted **rapid weight gain** (due to edema).
PE	VS: **tachycardia** (HR 102); **hypertension** (BP 160/100); no fever. PE: **eyelid and facial edema** (2+); funduscopy reveals **AV nicking;** hyperpigmentation of face (= CHLOASMA); chest clear; abdominal exam reveals term uterus; fetal tachycardia (HR 170); right upper quadrant tenderness; no hepatomegaly; **leg edema 3+;** brisk DTRs.
Labs	CBC: **increased hematocrit** (hemoconcentration); normal platelets (thrombocytopenia present in HELLP syndrome). **Hyperuricemia.** ABGs: mild acidosis. UA: marked **proteinuria.** LFTs: ALT and AST mildly elevated. Fibrinogen normal (may be decreased in associated abruptio placentae); PT/PTT normal. Lytes: normal. BUN and creatinine normal (may be increased in associated abruptio placentae).
Imaging	CXR: normal (no signs of aspiration pneumonia). CT-Head: cerebral edema; no focal lesion.
Pathogenesis	Preeclampsia refers to the triad of **hypertension** (increase in systolic blood pressure of > 30 mmHg or 15 mmHg diastolic above baseline level), **proteinuria,** and **nondependent edema** (> 5-lb gain/week) from the 20th week of pregnancy to one week postpartum. **Eclampsia refers to convulsions in a preeclamptic woman** that cannot be explained by any other etiology; it usually occurs in the prepartum period (75% of cases) but may occur up to 10 days postpartum (25% of cases). The etiology of preeclampsia is unknown, but women with hypertension, diabetes, collagen vascular, autoimmune, or renal disease prior to pregnancy are at increased risk

of developing preeclampsia and eclampsia.

Epidemiology   Occurs in approximately 1 in 2,000 pregnancies; more frequently seen among younger primigravidae of low socioeconomic groups and among Hispanics and blacks. Mortality is approximately 1%.

Management   Prevent and treat convulsions with slow administration of **magnesium sulfate** to prevent concomitant hypotension as a side effect. Magnesium toxicity is monitored by hourly measurement of DTRs, RR and depth, and urine output; toxicity can be counteracted by calcium gluconate. **Diazepam** may be used as an adjunctive therapy. If diastolic BP is > 110 mmHg, hydralazine, nifedipine, or labetalol may be used to keep diastolic BP around 90–100 mmHg. The definitive treatment of eclampsia is **early delivery** through either induction of labor or cesarean section.

Complications   **Fetal complications** include premature delivery, growth retardation, periventricular hemorrhage, necrotizing enterocolitis, and abruptio placentae. **Maternal complications** include airway obstruction, post-aspiration pneumonia, convulsions, fluid overload, hypoxia, acute renal failure, hepatic capsule rupture, and DIC. **FIRST AID 2** p. 245

Associated Diseases   ◘ **HELLP Syndrome** A variant of eclampsia; presents with Hemolysis, Elevated Liver enzymes, and Low Platelets; definitive treatment is delivery.

◘ **Hemolytic-Uremic Syndrome** Acute renal failure and microangiopathic hemolytic anemia, usually associated with bacterial (*E. coli, Shigella*) infection in children or following cancer chemotherapy (mitomycin); presents with fever, malaise, hypotension, ecchymoses, periorbital edema, and oliguria; schistocytes seen on PBS; no evidence of DIC (normal PT, PTT, fibrinogen); thrombocytopenia and elevated BUN and creatinine; treat with plasmapheresis, IV fluids and pressors as needed to prevent acute renal failure and hemodynamic compromise.

◘ **Thrombotic Thrombocytopenic Purpura** An idiopathic disease found in pregnant and HIV-positive patients and after exposure to antibiotics or estrogens; presents with episodic altered mental status, fever, renal dysfunction, petechiae over the chest and extremities, and fever; anemia, schistocytes on smear, low platelet count, and absent haptoglobin; treat with plasmapheresis.

ECLAMPSIA

ID/CC	A 32-year-old female presents with vaginal bleeding, **lightheadedness,** nausea, vomiting, and **fainting** after **sudden-onset left lower quadrant abdominal pain** two hours ago; the pain radiates to the scapular region and to the back (diaphragmatic irritation due to tubal rupture).
HPI	Several years ago, the patient was using an **IUD.** She has a history of **recurrent cervicitis and PID** due to *Neisseria gonorrhoeae* and had an appendectomy during childhood. Her **last menstrual period was 39 days ago,** but she states that she is regular and never misses a period.
PE	VS: **tachycardia (HR 110); orthostatic hypotension (BP 100/60 seated, 80/40 standing);** tachypnea (RR 24); low-grade fever. PE: marked **pallor; delayed capillary refill;** abdomen distended; **tender left iliac fossa** with voluntary guarding and **rebound tenderness; decreased bowel sounds;** pelvic exam reveals mild **tenderness on cervical motion** and soft, **tender left adnexal mass;** culdocentesis (diagnostic) reveals **nonclotting blood in cul-de-sac** (transvaginal ultrasound is replacing culdocentesis for diagnosis of ectopic pregnancy).
Labs	CBC: mild anemia (due to intraperitoneal bleeding); leukocytosis. Lytes: normal. Increased BUN. UA: normal. Serum **beta-hCG increased;** blood type O negative.
Imaging	[A] US-Pelvis: the ectopic gestation sac (1) is seen to be outside the empty uterus (2).
Pathogenesis	Implantation of the fertilized ovum outside the uterine cavity, usually in the ampullary region of the fallopian tubes, followed by the isthmus, fimbria, and interstitial portion (part of the tube that traverses the uterine wall). They may also implant in the cervix, the abdominal cavity, and the ovaries. The classic triad in ectopic pregnancy consists of **lower abdominal pain, amenorrhea, and vaginal bleeding,** but this triad is not always found. Interstitial pregnancy ruptures later with more profuse bleeding than other tubal pregnancies.
Epidemiology	Ectopic pregnancies have increased in incidence concomitantly with PID and are the **second leading cause of maternal mortality.** Hispanics and blacks have an increased incidence of ectopic pregnancy. Risk factors

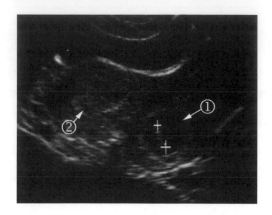

include **tubal ligation, PID** with scarring, **IUD** use, previous ectopic pregnancy, previous complicated appendicitis with peritonitis, endometriosis, multiparity, perimenopausal years, exposure to DES, and induction of ovulation.

Management

After hemodynamic stabilization (blood transfusion, etc.), a laparoscopy will confirm the diagnosis. An attempt at conservative surgery may be made laparoscopically by **salpingostomy** with removal of the product of conception or by **salpingectomy.** If the mother is Rh negative, then administer RhoGAM to prevent Rh isoimmunization. In the event of an unruptured ectopic pregnancy of < 3.5 cm, **methotrexate** may be given to induce abortion.

Complications

Risk of maternal exsanguination and death; increased incidence of future ectopic pregnancies and infertility due to tubal scarring.

Associated Diseases

■ **Adnexal Torsion** Associated with ovarian tumor or cyst; presents with abrupt, severe lower abdominal pain and mild fever; leukocytosis is often seen; laparoscopy is both diagnostic and therapeutic; complications include adnexal infarction.

■ **Pelvic Inflammatory Disease** A polymicrobial infection of the upper genital tract ascending from the lower genital tract, usually due to STDs caused by *Neisseria gonorrhoeae* and *Chlamydia trachomatis;* presents with lower abdominal pain and adnexal tenderness with vaginal discharge; leukocytosis with left shift; high vaginal and cervical swabs may yield organism; treat with cefoxitin and doxycycline; complications include tubo-ovarian abscess, peritonitis, ectopic pregnancy, and infertility.

◨ **Ruptured Corpus Luteum Cyst** Rupture of corpus luteum cysts; presents with unilateral abdominal pain and adnexal tenderness; negative beta-hCG; US may reveal evidence of ruptured cyst; treat with laparoscopic or open surgery to control bleeding.

ID/CC	A 27-year-old **primigravida** complains of persistent, severe vomiting and **excessive morning nausea and vomiting** of one month's duration.
HPI	Five weeks ago she tested positive on a urine pregnancy test. She has been amenorrheic for 12 weeks, and her **food and water intake has been markedly reduced** owing to persistent nausea. She shows evidence of **weight loss** of about seven pounds over the past month.
PE	VS: **tachycardia** (HR 105); **orthostatic hypotension.** PE: appears ill and moderately **dehydrated;** abdominal exam reveals fundal height to be at level of pelvic brim (12 weeks); fetal heart heard via doppler.
Labs	Serum hCG elevated (commensurate with period of gestation). Lytes: hyponatremia; hypokalemia. Abnormal TFTs (up to 60% of women with severe hyperemesis gravidarum have a transient elevation of T4). ABGs: **hypochloremic metabolic alkalosis.** UA: positive **ketones.** Further blood tests confirm **ketonemia.**
Imaging	US-Pelvis: single, live intrauterine 12-week gestation with positive fetal heart activity.
Pathogenesis	The cause of vomiting is thought to be high estrogen levels. Hyperemesis gravidarum is diagnosed when protracted vomiting is associated with dehydration and ketonuria.
Epidemiology	Half of all women, mostly primigravidae, complain of nausea and vomiting during early pregnancy. Hyperemesis gravidarum occurs in 4 out of 1,000 patients.
Management	Hospitalize and make NPO for 48 hours. Administer IV fluids (preferably glucose-saline); maintain electrolyte balance; if necessary, give antiemetics (prochlorperazine). After correction of acidosis, start gradual oral feeding. Other causes of hyperemesis must be ruled out.
Complications	In advanced cases, **renal and hepatic function may be compromised** (known as the toxemic phase of vomiting); in such cases and in cases that are resistant to intensive antiemetic therapy, **termination of pregnancy may be required.**

HYPEREMESIS GRAVIDARUM

Associated Diseases   ◼ **Hydatidiform Mole** Results from the fertilization of an empty ovum by normal sperm; presents with first-trimester bleeding, passage of vesicles per vagina, or hyperemesis; first-trimester preeclampsia (hypertension, edema, and proteinuria) is characteristic; beta-hCG markedly elevated; typical "snowstorm" pattern on pelvic US; requires immediate evacuation of uterine contents; complications include development of an invasive mole or choriocarcinoma.

ID/CC	A 31-year-old woman complains of **easy fatigability** and **lack of stamina for daily activities;** she has also had an unusual **urge to eat ice** (= PAGOPHAGIA) **and clay** (= PICA).
HPI	She is a **20-week primigravida** with an unremarkable medical history.
PE	VS: mild tachycardia (HR 105). PE: **pallor** of mucous membranes; fetal heart rate normal (140/min).
Labs	CBC: **microcytic, hypochromic** (MCHC < 30) anemia (may be normochromic or normocytic with concomitant folate deficiency); low hematocrit. **[A]** PBS: hypochromic and microcytic RBCs; poikilocytosis. **Low serum iron level; low transferrin saturation index** (< 16%); **increased TIBC; low ferritin level.** UA/Lytes: normal. Glucose normal.
Imaging	US-Abdomen: 20-week intrauterine pregnancy.
Pathogenesis	Anemia (Hct < 30 or Hb < 10) due to lack of iron resulting from diminished consumption, decreased absorption, increased demand (short interval between pregnancies), blood loss (hemorrhage), or a combination thereof. In pregnancy, iron absorption is usually increased (as opposed to folate) to offset increased demand. Because ferritin is the storage form of iron, **ferritin level is the test of choice in the diagnosis of iron deficiency** anemia.
Epidemiology	One-fifth of all pregnancies are associated with some degree of anemia, and iron deficiency is the most common cause of anemia in pregnancy (75%).
Management	Most pregnant patients receive supplemental iron in prenatal vitamin preparations, and this usually suffices for prophylaxis of overt anemia. If iron deficiency anemia is established, 325 mg of ferrous sulfate TID should be given. Administration of iron together with vitamin C increases absorption; taking it with antacids, calcium, or meals decreases absorption. Iron-dextran may be given IM if a patient cannot tolerate iron PO.
Complications	PO iron supplementation may cause black stools, epigastric discomfort, and constipation (often given with laxatives). IM iron-dextran administration may cause

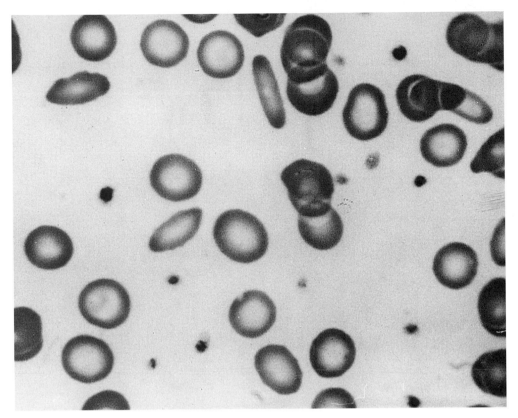

local pain or anaphylaxis.

Associated Diseases

◘ **Folate Deficiency** Folate is required for DNA/RNA synthesis; deficiency is most commonly associated with alcoholism, pregnancy, or medications (Bactrim, methotrexate, phenytoin); presents with fatigue, weakness, and nausea; anemia, hypersegmented PMNs, megaloblastic RBCs, and low RBC folate; treat with folic acid supplementation; folic acid is required for patients taking Bactrim or methotrexate.

◘ **Peptic Ulcer Disease** Due to a variety of factors, including *Helicobacter pylori* infection, emotional stress, abnormalities in the mucosa or in the secretion of acid, NSAID use, or cigarette smoking; presents with burning epigastric pain that is relieved by food; UGI endoscopy reveals evidence of peptic ulcer disease; endoscopically obtained biopsy and cytologic brushings may be used to confirm the diagnosis and to rule out gastric malignancy; evidence of *H. pylori* infection (ELISA for serologic detection of antibodies against *H. pylori,* breath urea test, histologic exam, culture and urease activity detection in endoscopic biopsy specimens); treat with ampicillin, clarithromycin, and metronidazole with H_2 blocker or proton pump inhibitor; complications include hemorrhage, perforation, gastric outlet obstruction, and gastric carcinoma.

◻ **Vitamin B12 Deficiency** Cofactor for DNA and myelin synthesis; deficiency is due to malabsorption (sprue, enteritis, *Diphyllobothrium latum* infection), absence of intrinsic factor (pernicious anemia), prolonged dietary deficiency (as in vegans), or terminal ileum disease; presents with anemia, degenerative changes in the spinal cord (especially the posterior columns and the corticospinal tracts), and peripheral neuropathies; hypersegmented PMNs, megaloblastic RBCs, and decreased serum vitamin B_{12}; treat the underlying disorder, IM vitamin B_{12}.

ID/CC	A **40-year-old multipara** at 36 weeks' gestation complains of **considerable vaginal bleeding.**
HPI	The bleeding is **bright red** but **painless** and of **sudden onset at rest.** The patient did not feel any uterine contractions, and the bleeding ceased after about an hour. For the past 28 weeks she has had **recurrent episodes of small amounts of vaginal bleeding;** these episodes were not preceded by trauma or intercourse, were painless, and stopped on their own. She is G7P6; the first four pregnancies were delivered vaginally and the last **two by cesarean section** (due to fetal distress and malpresentation).
PE	VS: normal. PE: **no tenderness** on abdominal exam; **uterus relaxed;** no contractions felt; **vaginal exam not performed** owing to risk of provoking bleeding.
Labs	CBC: normal. Blood grouped and cross-matched; **coagulation profile normal;** amniocentesis performed to **confirm fetal lung maturity** (lecithin/sphingomyelin ratio > 2:1).
Imaging	US-Abdomen: **total placenta previa** (placenta covering the cervical os) and a single live fetus in breech presentation and longitudinal lie; the biophysical profile (measure of fetal tone, movements, respiration, amniotic fluid index, fetal heart accelerations) is suggestive of fetal well-being.
Pathogenesis	No definite etiology is known. With US, placenta previa can be diagnosed early in pregnancy. **Asymptomatic placenta previa or low-lying placenta detected in the second trimester should be followed closely. Many migrate upward** and resolve as the uterus enlarges, while others remain in place; bleeding in a true placenta previa is physiologic and inevitable once the cervix begins to efface.
Epidemiology	Placenta previa occurs in about 0.5% of pregnancies; **predisposing factors** include **age > 35 years, multiparity, previous multiple abortions, previous cesarean sections, upper uterine cavity abnormalities, multiple gestation,** and **smoking.**
Management	Hospitalization; rule out local lesions of cervix and vagina; rule out abruptio placentae and refrain from

sexual intercourse. Indications for an emergent cesarean section in cases of placenta previa include persistent labor, bleeding > 500 mL, unstable bleeding requiring multiple transfusions, coagulation defects, documented fetal lung maturity, and a 36-week period of gestation. Before 36 weeks of gestation, steroids may be used to accelerate fetal lung maturity.

Complications

Maternal complications include hemorrhage, shock, death, or placenta accreta (abnormal implantation of chorionic villi into the myometrium; risk increases with previous cesarean section). **Fetal complications** include prematurity, blood loss, and death due to asphyxia or birth injury. **FIRST AID 2** p. 251

Associated Diseases

◘ **Placental Abruption** Premature separation of placental membranes from the myometrium secondary to maternal hemorrhage into the decidua basalis between the 20th week and birth; cocaine abuse is an important risk factor; presents with dark red vaginal bleeding, abdominal pain, DIC, and uterine rigidity (spasm); US shows hematoma, separation of the placental margin, and elevation of the chorioamnionic membrane; treat with close monitoring; severe disease requires IV fluids and pressors and emergent delivery.

ID/CC	A 30-year-old primigravida is brought to the emergency room with **continuous, painful vaginal bleeding.**
HPI	On admission, she began to **bleed from the IV site and from the nose.** She is calculated to be at 35 weeks' gestation and admits to **smoking** and **abusing cocaine;** she has also been **hypertensive** (cocaine induced) for the past month. She has had no prior episodes of similar vaginal bleeding but has a history of **physical abuse** by her husband.
PE	VS: **hypotension** (BP 100/60); **tachycardia** (HR 105). PE: looks extremely ill; epistaxis noted; abdominal exam reveals **tense uterus with marked tenderness; fetal heart audible but bradycardic** (HR 115); heavily blood-stained sanitary pad in place.
Labs	CBC/PBS: **thrombocytopenia;** fragmented RBCs. Coagulation profile reveals **prolonged clot retraction time, elevated fibrinogen degradation products, hypofibrinogenemia, prolonged PT/PTT and thrombin time,** and decreased anti-thrombin III and plasminogen.
Imaging	US-Abdomen: significant **placental abruption with a large retroplacental clot.**
Pathogenesis	Caused by premature separation of a normally implanted placenta before the third stage of labor. With intramyometrial infiltration of blood, the entire uterus appears matted and purplish (= COUVELAIRE UTERUS) and may lead to postpartum hemorrhage.
Epidemiology	The incidence of placental abruption is 1%; it is classified into marginal, partial, or total abruption and is the second most common cause of third-trimester bleeding. **Predisposing factors** include **preeclampsia, history of previous abruption, chronic hypertension, advanced maternal age, smoking and cocaine abuse, trauma,** and **sudden decrease in uterine volume** (such as that caused by ruptured membranes in polyhydramnios and after delivery of the first twin).
Management	**Fluid, blood, and cryoprecipitate** (for replacement of fibrinogen if bleeding complications occur) replacement; **immediate delivery** by cesarean section is indicated in cases of severe bleeding or fetal distress. Control

coagulation defects to limit bleeding during the postpartum period.

Complications   **Hemorrhagic shock** (sometimes due to concealed hemorrhage into a large retroplacental clot), **coagulopathy** (DIC occurs in 3% of severe abruptions), **ischemic necrosis of distant organs, postpartum hemorrhage, increased risk of recurrence in subsequent pregnancies,** and **fetal anemia.**

Associated Diseases   ◘ **Placenta Previa** Placental implantation over the cervical os; risk factors are prior cesarean section, multiparity, increasing age of the mother, fibroids, and previous placenta previa; presents as painless bright red vaginal bleeding in the third trimester; vaginal examination is contraindicated; US shows abnormal implantation; treat with emergent cesarean delivery to prevent massive hemorrhage.

ID/CC	A 28-year-old woman presents to a family clinic with **weight gain** and **difficulty breathing.**
HPI	Her last menstrual period was 24 weeks ago. She had a normal full-term pregnancy and delivered a healthy male baby vaginally three years ago; she has no history of any abortions or stillbirths. She has no history of diabetes or hypertension, and her blood group is B positive. Her current pregnancy was diagnosed at home via urine testing, and she sought no prenatal care.
PE	VS: tachycardia (HR 105); normal BP; tachypnea (RR 24). PE: no pallor, icterus, or pedal edema; abdominal exam reveals markedly distended abdomen; **fundal height corresponds to 32 weeks'** gestation (calculated at 24 weeks); **fluid thrill** palpable in all directions; **distant and feeble fetal heart sounds** audible.
Labs	**Serum alpha-fetoprotein (AFP)** (ideally should have been done at 15–20 weeks of gestation) **elevated; screening test for gestational diabetes negative** (polyhydramnios is frequently associated with maternal diabetes).
Imaging	US-Abdomen: polyhydramnios **(amniotic fluid index > > 20)** and **anencephalic fetus.**
Pathogenesis	Polyhydramnios is diagnosed on the basis of **an amniotic fluid index of > 20.** Although its exact cause is not known, it is strongly associated with **uniovular twin pregnancy,** in which the hydramnios affects only one amniotic sac (usually the upper); **neural tube defects** such as **anencephaly** and **spina bifida;** congenital esophageal defects such as tracheoesophageal fistula or pyloric stenosis; **maternal diabetes** and **cardiac** or **renal disease;** and **chorioangioma of the placenta,** a rare tumor that generally presents with an acute polyhydramnios. **Polyhydramnios is invariably present when there is an open defect allowing free communication with the CSF.**
Epidemiology	Affects 0.4% of all pregnancies. The defect varies from anencephaly, encephalocele, and meningomyelocele to spina bifida.
Management	Frequent US examinations; perform therapeutic amniocentesis in the presence of maternal respiratory

compromise/marked uterine distention. Tocolysis if premature labor ensues; deliver if fetus is mature. To detect neural tube defects, **maternal serum AFP is recommended as a routine screening prenatal test at 15–20 weeks of pregnancy;** an elevated level of maternal serum AFP is followed with amniotic fluid AFP, acetylcholinesterase levels, and an obstetric US to confirm the diagnosis. **Folic acid supplementation** is recommended for the next pregnancy to reduce the risk of neural tube defects.

Complications   N/A

Associated Diseases   N/A

ID/CC	A 30-year-old woman complains of **cessation of menses** (= AMENORRHEA) for two months along with a feeling of **fullness in her breasts, early-morning nausea, and vomiting** (pregnancy).
HPI	The patient is the mother of a child who was born of a normal vaginal delivery three years ago; four months ago she had an **IUD** (progestasert) inserted.
PE	VS: normal. PE: **IUD in place** with **strings visible** on speculum exam.
Labs	CBC/Lytes: normal. **Pregnancy test positive.** UA: normal; urine culture and sensitivity normal.
Imaging	US-Pelvis: IUD inside uterus; product of conception implanted on the uterine fundus.
Pathogenesis	The IUD is one of the most effective methods of reversible contraception (failure rate is < 2% per six years of use). IUDs prevent the implantation of the fertilized ovum by creating a hostile endometrium (subclinical endometritis) via an inflammatory response to the foreign body; they also exert a spermicidal action through increased phagocytosis. IUDs may contain copper (spermicidal) or progesterone (direct action on the endometrium; needs to be changed annually) for added effectiveness. They are inserted during menstruation to avoid pregnancy. **Advantages** are the ability to confer **long-term (up to 10 years) contraception** with only periodic checkups and obviating the need for patient compliance with medications. **Contraindications** include pregnancy, previous septic abortion (within three months), gynecologic infections, abnormal Pap smears, uterine malformations, and Wilson's disease (with copper-containing IUDs).
Epidemiology	Of all pregnancies that occur with IUDs, 1 in 20 are septic. The rate of spontaneous abortion may be increased up to 40% for women with an IUD in place. Given this, the device needs to be removed if continuation of pregnancy is desired. IUDs are not associated with an increased risk of congenital malformations. After an IUD has been removed, 90% of patients not using other forms of contraception become

pregnant within a year.

Management   If the patient wants to continue the pregnancy and strings are visible, the IUD must be gently removed. If the strings are not visible and no part of the IUD is located near the cervical os for easy grasping, the device may be left in place with careful periodic observation.

Complications   Perforation of the uterine fundus during insertion (1:2,000), spontaneous expulsion (10%; highest incidence during the first year after placement), increased menstrual flow and intermenstrual bleeding, dysmenorrhea (sometimes incapacitating), pregnancy, ectopic pregnancy (5% of IUD-related pregnancies), actinomycotic adnexal abscess, and increased incidence of PID (more so if relations are not monogamous).

Associated Diseases   N/A

ID/CC	A 30-year-old woman presents with **fever,** malaise, and **lower abdominal pain** five days **following a cesarean section.**
HPI	Her **lochia (uterine discharge) has become purulent** and is particularly **foul-smelling.** She does not complain of breast discomfort, dysuria, cough, or any painful injection site; the baby is healthy.
PE	VS: tachycardia (HR 110); mild tachypnea (RR 20); normal BP; fever (38.9 C). PE: breast examination normal; chest exam normal; **uterine tenderness;** lochia staining pad is purulent and foul-smelling; surgical wound clean, dry, and intact.
Labs	CBC: **leukocytosis.** UA: trace albumin. **High vaginal swab was stained and cultured;** Gram stain reveals gram-positive cocci and gram-negative bacilli; culture shows **group B streptococci,** *E. coli*, **and anaerobic peptostreptococci;** blood culture is sterile.
Imaging	N/A
Pathogenesis	Caused by normal bacteria in the vaginal flora, which may become pathogenic during the puerperium (due to alteration in normal defenses) or from exogenous pathogens. Diagnosis is clinical with findings of fever (>100.4 F or 38 C for at least 2 of the first 10 days of the puerperium, excluding the first 24 hours), elevated WBC count, and uterine tenderness.
Epidemiology	Risk factors include **early rupture of the membranes, prolonged labor, numerous vaginal examinations, use of internal monitoring devices, and instrumental** and **operative deliveries such as cesarean section.**
Management	Antibiotic treatment includes a combination of an **aminoglycoside** (for gram-negative bacilli), a **third-generation cephalosporin** (for gram-positive and resistant gram-negative coverage), and **metronidazole** (for anaerobic coverage); heparin is administered for septic pelvic thrombophlebitis. In addition to antibiotics, **D&C may be required** to remove retained products of conception.
Complications	**Sepsis,** acute renal failure, septic **pelvic thrombophlebitis,** shock and death.

ID/CC	A 20-year-old college student is brought to the ER after being found in an alley.
HPI	The patient does not speak, and her clothes are torn and bloody.
PE	VS: tachycardia (HR 110); normal BP; tachypnea (RR 20); no fever. PE: one **laceration** on scalp with dried blood; several **scratches** on face; **right eye swollen** shut and ecchymotic; lip swollen; **two front teeth missing;** chest and arms show **fingernail scratches** and several **ecchymoses and hematomas;** inner thighs reveal streaks of dried blood and semen; vulva swollen and excoriated; small branches and leaves stuck to skin of posterior legs and buttocks.
Labs	CBC: normal. RPR/HIV negative. UA: mild hematuria. Samples from throat, anus, and vagina sent for Gram stain and gonococcal and chlamydia culture; pregnancy test negative.
Imaging	CXR: normal.
Pathogenesis	Rape constitutes an **expression of power and aggression** on the part of the perpetrator, who uses sexual acts to threaten and hurt the victim. Rape involves the **illegal penetration of any orifice in the body by hand, penis, or object.**
Epidemiology	Rape is underreported; approximately half of all cases are reported. Rape may be committed by an acquaintance or spouse; **50% of rapists are known to the victim.** The vast majority of victims are women, but the number of male victims is on the rise.
Management	Recognize the great **psychological trauma** of the patient. Shame, remorse, guilt, fear, and anger are initially experienced, and these are best dealt with by trained counselors. A **respectful** and **noncritical attitude** will be most beneficial to the victim. A detailed history should also be taken, including relevant obstetrical and gynecologic data such as last date of coitus (to aid in semen analysis), last menstrual period, pregnancy status, and prior STDs; a physical examination should then be completed for forensic purposes. Particulate matter should be collected as evidence (fingernail scrapings, pubic hair combings, dirt,

pieces of clothing leaves). A Wood's light will allow semen to be visualized. Obtain samples from the mouth, anus, and vagina, and record the percentage of motile sperm. Cultures for gonococcus and chlamydia should be obtained as well as a Pap smear, a *Trichomonas vaginalis* wet prep, VDRL, HIV, and pregnancy tests. Ceftriaxone and doxycycline/azithromycin may be given for the prevention of gonorrhea and chlamydia. Treat wounds with local care and tetanus prophylaxis, and vaccinate against hepatitis B. Pregnancy prophylaxis may be given with 0.5 mg of norgestrel/0.05 mg ethinylestradiol, two tabs PO in the ER and two tabs PO 12 hours afterward.

Complications

The **rape trauma syndrome** consists of immediate and chronic phases. In the immediate phase, a victim may experience severe mood swings and feelings of anger, guilt, disbelief, and denial. In the chronic phase, a victim may experience nightmares and relationship difficulties. Other complications include gonorrhea, syphilis, HIV, and pregnancy.

Associated Diseases

N/A

ID/CC	A 40-year-old woman who underwent **tubal ligation 10 years ago requests reversal;** she has remarried and now wants a child.
HPI	Her menstrual periods are regular, and her last delivery was 10 years ago.
PE	VS: normal. PE: small Pfannenstiel incision (tubal ligation); pelvic and rectal exam normal.
Labs	CBC/Lytes/UA: normal. PT/PTT normal.
Imaging	CXR/KUB: normal. US-Pelvis: normal uterus.
Pathogenesis	Although tubal ligation is **definitive,** many patients may request reversal. Tubal ligation is performed by open surgery or by laparoscopy and involves a variety of techniques, including the Pomeroy operation (a loop of tube is tied with absorbable suture, a portion is removed, and the ends separate with a gap once the suture absorbs), fimbriectomy, spring clips (= HULKA CLIPS), Silastic bands, and electrocauterization.
Epidemiology	Tubal ligation is performed twice as frequently as vasectomy. Laparoscopic tubal ligation has a failure rate of up to 1 in 100, whereas the Pomeroy operation has a failure rate of 1 in 500; all methods taken together show a failure rate of 1%. The pregnancy rate after tubal ligation decreases with time after the operation, but the ectopic pregnancy rate remains the same; 30% of the pregnancies that occur after tubal ligation are ectopic.
Management	**Reanastomosis** may be tried with microsurgical techniques. Tubal reconstruction does not guarantee the return of reproductive potential and has an increased risk of **ectopic pregnancy. In vitro fertilization** or **artificial insemination** may be an option.
Complications	Bleeding, infection, and visceral injury.
Associated Diseases	N/A

ID/CC	A 35-year-old female complains of **infrequent menstrual bleeding** occurring at > 40-day intervals (= OLIGOMENORRHEA) coupled with **cold intolerance, coarse hair,** episodes of sweating with lightheadedness and weakness (due to hypoglycemia), **weight loss** (6 kg in three months), and a feeling of constant **fatigue.**
HPI	The patient suffered an **abruptio placentae** seven years ago (average delay for onset of symptoms) with **severe bleeding** followed by **hypovolemic shock.** She had **failure of lactation** and quick breast involution (most common presenting sign) following the pregnancy. She had **persistent amenorrhea** for a year.
PE	VS: **hypotension** (BP 100/50); tachycardia (HR 104); no fever. PE: dry skin; **coarse hair;** slow speech; thick tongue; periorbital swelling; **delayed relaxation phase of DTRs,** especially ankle (due to hypothyroidism); **hyperpigmentation** of palms and buccal mucosa; **lack of axillary and pubic hair** (due to adrenal insufficiency); vaginal exam reveals atrophic mucosa (due to lack of gonadotropin).
Labs	CBC: normocytic, normochromic anemia; lymphocytosis; eosinophilia (due to adrenal insufficiency). **Low prolactin and cortisol; low T4 and estradiol levels; low ACTH and TSH; low gonadotropins; failure of growth hormone to increase** (to > 7 ng/mL) **after insulin-induced hypoglycemia** (to < 40 mg/dL or to 50% of blood glucose level) (most common laboratory abnormality in hypopituitarism); IV TRH fails to stimulate TSH and prolactin secretion. Lytes: hyponatremia; hyperkalemia (due to decreased aldosterone). ABGs: metabolic acidosis (due to adrenal insufficiency).
Imaging	MR-Head: the sella turcica fails to show neoplastic or infiltrative involvement.
Pathogenesis	A result of **ischemia following severe obstetric hemorrhage with necrosis of the pituitary** gland. It is frequently associated with abruptio placentae and coagulopathy. After destruction of the pituitary gland, growth hormone, gonadotropic, thyroid, adrenal, and lactation (prolactin) functions are lost. Symptoms may be delayed for months or years.

51.   **SHEEHAN'S SYNDROME**

Epidemiology	N/A
Management	**Thyroid, estrogen,** and **corticosteroid replacement.** Rule out pituitary tumor. Early detection is key.
Complications	Infertility, metabolic derangements, and addisonian crisis.
Associated Diseases	◻ **Hypopituitarism** Causes include adenoma of the anterior pituitary in adults and craniopharyngioma in children; presents with cold intolerance, hypotension, bitemporal hemianopsia, and testicular atrophy; low FSH, LH, TSH, and ACTH; XR shows widening of the sella turcica; treat by hormone replacement and surgical resection of tumor.

ID/CC	A newborn is evaluated for **congenital malformations.**
HPI	The mother is a **chronic smoker** but does not abuse alcohol or other drugs; she had no skin rashes or viral prodrome during pregnancy. Routine prenatal tests, including rubella antibody titers, were negative. The baby had a **low birth weight.**
PE	Baby appears **small for age; microcephaly** and **cleft lip** present.
Labs	N/A
Imaging	N/A
Pathogenesis	Effects are due to a direct fetoplacental effect of nicotine and its metabolites as well as to reduced fetal oxygenation.
Epidemiology	N/A
Management	Strongly **discourage cigarette smoking,** especially during subsequent pregnancies.
Complications	Complications include increased risk of **low birth weight, microcephaly,** cleft lip and palate, **placenta previa,** placental abruption, **preeclampsia,** and premature and prolonged rupture of membranes. Maternal cigarette smoking is one of the most common **preventable risk factors for late fetal demise.** There is a long-term relationship between smoking during pregnancy and retarded intellectual development of offspring.
Associated Diseases	◼ **Fetal Alcohol Syndrome** The leading cause of fetal malformations in the U.S.; presents with microcephaly, growth retardation, and mental retardation; CXR reveals cardiomegaly; no specific treatment; complications include cardiac septal defects.

SMOKING DURING PREGNANCY

ID/CC	A 30-year-old primigravida at 32 weeks' gestation complains of **swelling around the eyes and over her feet.**
HPI	She initiated prenatal care at 12 weeks' gestation. **Ultrasound at 18 weeks revealed a twin pregnancy;** subsequent ultrasound at 24 weeks revealed the presence of **hydramnios.** No congenital malformations were found in either fetus.
PE	VS: **tachycardia** (HR 110); **hypertension** (BP 140/90); mild tachypnea (RR 20); no fever. PE: **pedal edema; fundal height corresponds to 36 weeks** (more than calculated period of gestation); multiple fetal parts felt; two fetal hearts heard by two different examiners; rates differed by at least 10 beats/minute.
Labs	CBC: normal. UA: **proteinuria + +**; 24-hour urine collection contained 900 mg of protein. **Serum uric acid elevated.**
Imaging	US-Abdomen: gross **polyhydramnios; the first twin is vertex, second is breech;** on the basis of measurements of head circumference, abdominal circumference, and biparietal diameter, the second twin **reveals evidence of intrauterine growth retardation.**
Pathogenesis	**Monozygotic twins with monochorionic placenta can develop twin-twin (= FETO-FETAL) transfusion syndrome.** Vascular communication between the twins can result in one fetus with hypervolemia, cardiomegaly, glomerulotubular hypertrophy, ascites, and edema and the other with hypovolemia, growth restriction, and oligohydramnios.
Epidemiology	Without assisted fertility, the incidence of twin gestation is about 1 in 80, with 30% monozygotic; the incidence has increased with assisted fertility, both with induction of ovulation with clomiphene and with in vitro fertilization where multiple embryo transfer is undertaken.
Management	Concordant twins should be evaluated for growth with US every four weeks beginning at 24 weeks. At 36 weeks, patients should be evaluated with non-stress tests and biophysical profiles twice weekly. Discordant twins are tested more often and are delivered at onset of lung

TWIN PREGNANCY

maturity or fetal distress.

Complications Complications include **preterm labor, placenta previa, cord prolapse, postpartum hemorrhage, gestational diabetes, polyhydramnios, preeclampsia, and anemia.** The fetuses are at an increased risk of congenital malformations, low birth weight, and malpresentation.

Associated Diseases N/A

From the authors of *Underground Clinical Vignettes*

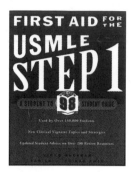

A true classic used by over 200,000 students around the world. The '99 edition features details on the new computerized test, new color plates and thoroughly updated high-yield facts and book reviews. Bi-directional links with the *Underground Clinical Vignettes Step 1* series. ISBN 0-8385-2612-8.

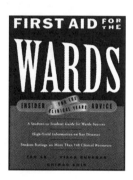

This high-yield student-to-student guide is designed to help students make the transition from the basic sciences to the hospital wards and succeed on their clinical rotations. The book features an orientation to the hospital environment, tips on being an effective and efficient junior medical student, student-proven advice tailored to each core rotation, a database of high-yield clinical facts, and recommendations for clinical pocket books, texts, and references. ISBN 0-8385-2595-4.

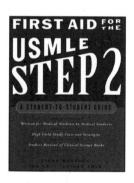

This entirely rewritten second edition now follows in the footsteps of *First Aid for the USMLE Step 1*. Features an exam preparation guide geared to the new computerized test, basic science and clinical high-yield facts, color plates and ratings of USMLE Step 2 books and software. Bi-directional links with the *Underground Clinical Vignettes Step 2* series.

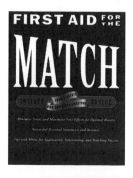

This top rated (5 stars, *Doody Review*) student-to-student guide helps medical students effectively and efficiently navigate the residency application process, helping them make the most of their limited time, money, and energy. The book draws on the advice and experiences of successful student applicants as well as residency directors. Also featured are application and interview tips tailored to each specialty, successful personal statements and CVs with analyses, current trends, and common interview questions with suggested strategies for responding. ISBN 0-8385-2596-2.

The *First Aid* series by Appleton & Lange...the review book leader.
Available through your local health sciences bookstore !